MW00653242

Praise for **Sober*ful***

"Veronica gets it, and this book is the missing piece for people who want to live a vibrant life without alcohol. If you're questioning your relationship with alcohol in any way, this is the book you need right now. In straight-talking chapters filled with compassionate advice and accessible tools, Veronica delivers a message that is both hopeful and actionable."

LAURA MCKOWEN
bestselling author of *We Are the Luckiest: The Surprising Magic of a Sober Life*

"I love Veronica Valli's new book for its clarity, approachability, and basic common sense. Persuasive without being preachy in the slightest, this is a fabulous book and essential reading for anyone wanting to kick the booze."

LUCY ROCCA
founder of Soberistas, coauthor of *The Sober Revolution: Women Calling Time on Wine O'Clock*, and author of *Glass Half Full: A Positive Journey to Living Alcohol-Free*

"Valli posits a new and different narrative about the perception of alcohol, its pervasiveness in our culture, and how it has historically (and systematically) affected our behaviors and belief systems. *Soberful* suggests that we can change our misguided beliefs about the benefits of alcohol by revising our perspective, learning a new language, and realizing the power of connection. Valli's Five Pillars of Sustainable Sobriety provide the inspiration and structure necessary for us to discover the root of the problem and attack it with gusto."

LAURIE DHUE
National Recovery Advocate and former CNN,
MSNBC, and Fox News anchor

"Veronica Valli has written a comprehensive guide to getting sober. This simple, straightforward program will help anyone who applies it. Based on her years of experience as a therapist and coach, Veronica takes the reader through a process that will not just get them sober but help them live an empowered, expansive life. Highly recommended."

SHERRY GABA, LCSW
coauthor of *Love Smacked* and *Infinite Recovery* and the
go-to expert on VH1's *Celebrity Rehab*

"For those of us who happened upon the 'cyber-sober sphere' in and around 2010, Veronica Valli was already a bit of a legend in the recovery blogging space. A woman in long-term recovery herself, Veronica has always excelled at delivering a no-nonsense, inclusive, and easy-to-understand message to people either exploring their relationship with alcohol or trying to save their lives from alcohol destruction. Being a skilled therapist helps her hammer home the simple truth—life is better when we show up for it fully present. This book is a distillation of decades of Veronica's work and is a welcome addition to the burgeoning literature devoted to recovery from behavioral health issues."

DAWN NICKEL, PHD
founder of SHE RECOVERS® Foundation

"*Soberful*, the new book by my friend Veronica Valli, is a discussion of the great big sober secret: you can get to the land of fun, excitement, belonging, connection, relaxation, rewards, and romance without alcohol. Sober does not mean somber; it simply means awake to all that life has to offer. This book will walk you through the process, answer questions, and open your eyes to new possibilities."

MARY GAUTHIER
Grammy®-nominated American folk singer
and author of *Saved by a Song*

"With over 21 years of sobriety, Veronica is an oracle of all things alcohol-free and shows that happy and sustainable sobriety is not only possible but wonderful too."

MILLIE GOOCH
founder of the Sober Girl Society
and author of *The Sober Girl Society Handbook*

"Recovery is a lifestyle, and Veronica Valli has established herself as a leading ambassador of this beautiful lifestyle. *Soberful* provides readers with practical solutions for trying on a new pair of glasses in their approach to life, addressing many of the common fears and roadblocks that people face along the way. I am proud to add *Soberful* as the latest book to my recovery library, and I will be enthusiastically recommending it to my clients, students, and members of my recovery circles."

JAMIE MARICH, PHD
author of *Trauma and the 12 Steps: An Inclusive Guide to Enhancing Recovery* and founder of the Institute for Creative Mindfulness and the Dancing Mindfulness approach to expressive arts therapy

"*Soberful* is an insightful read for anyone seeking change in their relationship with alcohol. Veronica Valli's personal and professional expertise combine to give her a level of compassion and wisdom that informs and resonates."

JEAN MCCARTHY
author of *UnPickled Holiday Survival Guide* and *The Ember Ever There* and host of *The Bubble Hour* podcast

"*Soberful* is a great road map from a sober legend who knows the pitfalls and the joys of the sober path, which gently and expertly guides you through the transitions of early sobriety to a place of happy and sustainable sobriety. This book is going to help so many people to embrace a sober and full life."

KATE BAILY
coauthor of *Love Yourself Sober*

"In *Soberful*, author Veronica Valli offers a gentle self-accepting path forward to live the life you crave, one that substances have robbed you of feeling you actually deserve. The practical steps in this book to help you rediscover a meaningful sober life make this an indispensable guide for those who want to take the first step and also for those who work in the recovery field."

ALINA FRANK
cofounder of EFT Tapping Training Institute and author of *How to Want Sex Again*

"A must-read for anyone who is concerned about their own drinking or someone else's. Wise, simple, practical advice written with compassion and genuine concern."

JOE SCHRANK
clinical social worker, founder of The Fix,
and executive editor of *The Small Bow*

"Veronica is the voice of wisdom we all need in the ever-growing jungle of alcohol addiction and recovery books. She is an accomplished professional with years of education, training, and practice, who also has personal experience living a healthy, vibrant life without alcohol for twenty-one years. If you are questioning your relationship with alcohol, this book offers you clear guidance for making sense of this relationship. With the Five Pillars of Sustainable Sobriety, Veronica has developed a sustainable program for shifting your mindset, doing the work, and truly transforming your life."

LYNN MATTI
clinical psychotherapist, addiction specialist,
and host of *The Sober Therapist* podcast

"Refreshing, hopeful, and compassionate. Veronica has a gift for breaking down the true key to lasting sobriety and creating logical guidelines that make achieving it possible for anyone who reads this book. No overwhelming science jargon, just understandable and truthful concepts to help you get where you want to go."

KELLY FITZGERALD JUNCO
founder of Sober Señorita

soberful

sober*ful*

UNCOVER
A SUSTAINABLE,
FULFILLING LIFE
FREE OF
ALCOHOL

VERONICA VALLI

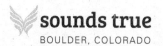
sounds true
BOULDER, COLORADO

Sounds True
Boulder, CO 80306

Published 2022

Book design by Linsey Dodaro

The wood used to produce this book is from Forest Stewardship
Council (FSC) certified forests, recycled materials, or controlled wood.

Printed in Canada

BK06263

Library of Congress Cataloging-in-Publication Data

Names: Valli, Veronica, author.
Title: Soberful : uncover a sustainable, fulfilling life free of alcohol / by
  Veronica Valli.
Description: Boulder, CO : Sounds True, 2022. | Includes bibliographical
  references.
Identifiers: LCCN 2021014780 (print) | LCCN 2021014781 (ebook) | ISBN
  9781683648291 (hardback) | ISBN 9781683648307 (ebook)
Subjects: LCSH: Temperance. | Alcoholics—Rehabilitation. |
  Alcoholism—Treatment.
Classification: LCC HV5060 .V25 2022 (print) | LCC HV5060 (ebook) | DDC
  616.88/106—dc23
LC record available at https://lccn.loc.gov/2021014780
LC ebook record available at https://lccn.loc.gov/2021014781

10 9 8 7 6 5 4 3 2 1

This book is dedicated to all those who
seek a glorious alcohol-free life.

Beneath the surface we are connected.

KAE TEMPEST, *On Connection*

CONTENTS

Before you stop drinking:

The information in this book is for educational purposes only and is not meant to replace any advice from a health-care professional. Please consult your health-care professional before you give up alcohol. Withdrawal from alcohol can be life threatening and even fatal.

FOREWORD

have never written a foreword before. I have never even thought about the process or what it would involve. I never thought I would have to give thought or consideration on how to craft a foreword.

This is a first for me.

I have, though, been working in the field of problem drug and alcohol use for thirty-five years. I have managed and run rehabilitation facilities, developed novel approaches to the issue of recovery, and helped people like Russell Brand get sober—a fact he has graciously acknowledged in public.

I have also worked with Veronica Valli before. I gave her her first internship, and I have therefore followed Veronica's career with interest—at times, awe—for the amount of work she has put into honing her skills and knowledge. It was her idea to start a podcast that she called *Soberful*, and she asked me to join her. I had never participated in a podcast before, let alone shared the platform with someone. It was Veronica's push that taught me that even an "old dog" could learn new tricks, could push the boundaries of what they thought possible. The *Soberful* podcast has grown and grown. I owe Veronica for the opportunity she gave me to end my career as part of a recovery tool that I am immensely proud of. If *Soberful* is my career swan song, I will be content and happy. What she taught me is that anything is possible even if at first you don't believe you can achieve the task offered to you.

There are a lot of books in the genre of "quit lit." There are even more people working in the field of self-help and personal growth. Where once there were few, there are now many. But not many are as qualified and experienced as Veronica is.

In the time I have been working, I have seen many changes in approach, style, and methodology. I have seen certain styles come and go. Therapeutic gurus come in and out of favor. I have watched as new methods of intervention become the model of the year, or decade. It is a field of endeavor that is constantly on the move.

There are, though, two things that remain consistent. First, there are many people out there who are struggling to know how to deal with a developing alcohol problem. They have tried doing it on their own, dabbled with various attempts at control, and at some point find themselves hoping, as you do now, that some guidance and advice will help them out of the darkness into a lighter and better life.

The second constant is that the most successful help and support comes from people who understand, empathize, and give clear, nonjudgmental support and encouragement, people who can get to the heart of an issue quickly, simply, and in a way that demonstrates a genuine desire to see people reach their full potential.

This book matters. It talks directly to those searching for answers. It is accessible and does not talk down to the reader or baffle them with science. It is bursting with precisely the sort of advice you have been looking for. And it does so because it is written by someone with professional skill and expertise, someone I have been proud to work alongside. I hope that this book and the heart and passion of Veronica's words will help you put your past behind you and show you that a better, different life is not just achievable but eminently desirable too.

Chip Somers, psychotherapist and cohost of the *Soberful* podcast

Introduction

I know you have been thinking about this for a while. You've seen a few posts on social media; maybe you've even known a friend or two who has decided to stop drinking. A few people getting sober, in itself, may not seem revolutionary. But the fact that they are sharing this information publicly, with strangers, is a very big deal.

For too long in our alcohol-saturated world, being a non-drinker has been a shocking and taboo subject. Becoming alcohol-free was nothing to be proud of—quite the opposite. To say that you don't drink or have stopped drinking is to be greeted with looks of shock, disbelief, and confusion, and maybe sometimes with quiet envy. Adults drink alcohol; this is just a fact, which is why we struggle so much with the idea of quitting. Because who would give up drinking when it brings us so much? Alcohol is everywhere. It's impossible to avoid, and we harness it to every social situation we can think of, every celebration, every rite of passage. It is a ubiquitous substance that follows us through life.

Over the years I have noticed that more and more people are realizing that their relationship with alcohol no longer makes sense. And they are experiencing consequences they don't want. Some of us are, in fact, drinking far more than is good for our mental, emotional, and physical health.

When we use alcohol to socialize, to feel less lonely, to help us belong, it's because we believe alcohol is our friend. Our culture promotes alcohol as beneficial and deliberately obscures all of its costs and consequences.

These days the line has blurred, and we don't know what constitutes an alcohol problem and what doesn't. I think most people define a person with an alcohol problem as someone who drinks 24/7, who has vodka for breakfast and passes out drunk every night. And if you are not that, then you must not have a problem. We breathe a sigh of relief and think, *My drinking is not that bad. I should be able to manage it if I just try hard enough.* But things still don't feel right, do they? You can dismiss the thoughts, but they keep creeping back. And you still wonder if something is up with your drinking.

It's hard to admit, isn't it? Because if you admit that you may (not definitely, just, you know, possibly) have an issue with alcohol then lots of scary words flood into your mind like *boring*, *teetotaler*, *dull*, and *missing out*. At first glance, sobriety doesn't seem to have much to recommend itself. When you are surrounded by messages reinforcing how much fun alcohol is, why would you stop? But people are stopping, and not just those who recognize that alcohol is causing problems in their life—people who are electing not to drink as a lifestyle choice. Because they can see that alcohol is not necessary to fun, excitement, belonging, connection, relaxation, rewards, and romance. It's like a mini sober revolution is taking place.

If you have come to this book because you know it's time to quit, I want you to know I was in your shoes twenty years ago. When we think about giving up alcohol, we also believe we have to give up all the wonderful things that go with it. And this is why quitting alcohol feels hard at the beginning. You're going to have to give up fun, friends, connection, being part of a group. What about celebrations, nights out, dating, sex, all those wonderful things? Surely if you quit alcohol, you will be quitting those things too? Imagine how empty, dull, and boring your life is going to be.

Well, what if I told you that none of those things were true? That in fact you had been lied to. Sure, alcohol can accompany lots of fun and adventures, but you don't need alcohol to have the fun and adventures. In fact, just the opposite. What we are discussing here is a question of *perception*. And I want you to hold on to the thought that your current perception of alcohol and sobriety may be faulty.

***

At some point some people cross a line and suddenly their relationship with alcohol no longer makes sense. But do you know where that line is? How would you know if you had crossed it?

I can tell you that the line is the point where drinking costs us more than just money; it's when we start behaving in ways that are out of alignment with our values and beliefs. Have you felt pressured to drink when you just don't want to, because you want to be accepted and to fit in? Have you ever felt ashamed because of something you said or did when you were drunk? What about the people you love? Would your kids, spouse, neighbors, or friends describe your drinking as "fun"?

It's tough for us to know when our drinking is costing us more than we want to pay. The line has been deliberately blurred, so much so that most of us don't realize when we have crossed it. Abnormal drinking has been normalized. Our culture supports it. When you see yourself reflected in everyone else around you, why would you question what is normal?

The biggest reason that most people have for not quitting alcohol is the belief that if they don't drink, they will be "missing out." What they are going to miss out on is often ill-defined, yet it is a strong and powerful force that either pushes people to continue drinking long past the point of fun or to put enormous effort into trying to moderate, with little success. It is the fear of potential loss that motivates these thoughts. So, we plod on with dogged determination to find a way to drink alcohol but face no consequences, because the idea of not drinking at all is too much for us to cope with.

I see you. I know you are at that point. And I'm going to let you into a delicious and wonderful secret. Despite everything you have been told and all that you believe, a life without alcohol is more fun, more fulfilling, more connected, and more expansive than drinking ever was. You may not believe me right now, or you may be telling yourself the story, *Yes, I can see it would be for you, but I'm different.* But I promise that you and I are not different at all and that an incredible sober life is possible for you as well.

This book is not about persuading you to stop drinking. Instead, I want to introduce you to what is possible if you change your relationship with alcohol. What I lay out in the subsequent chapters is a program for people to do the deeper personal development work all human beings have to do. Because it's not just about stopping alcohol, it's about transformation at a much deeper level. Maybe you have listened to all of the podcasts, read all the "quit lit," and have been trying to stop but feel like you are floundering a bit. The reason for that is you don't have a program. A method to follow that gives you the support to say no to alcohol and grow into the person you are capable of being. The five pillars of sustainable sobriety that I provide in this book will give you that support.

I see more and more people realizing this, putting down the booze, and walking toward a life that they had no idea was possible. It's a life full of possibility and hope, connection and meaning, purpose and joy. It's a life filled with more, not less. Just let me show you how getting there can be easier than you think.

Welcome to a Soberful life.

PART ONE

Does My Relationship with
Alcohol Make Sense?

CHAPTER 1

How Do I Know If I Should Stop or Not?

Most clients who reach out to me are aware that something is wrong in their lives, but they're not convinced the problem is alcohol. Most initially want to become "social" or "normal" drinkers again. A few are open to a period of abstinence, but nearly all are horrified by the idea of never drinking again. That feels like a fate worse than death.

But on some level, they know that their relationship with alcohol doesn't add up anymore. And I think to some degree they also know that their struggle is masking deeper issues. We have an inkling that we use alcohol to cope with feelings and emotions we couldn't otherwise manage.

I want you to know that no one ends up in front of me by accident. You are not reading this book by accident. I've never had anyone reach out to me via my website, my Soberful Facebook group, or my programs and thought to myself, *Blimey, what are they doing here? They are absolutely fine.* If they think about alcohol enough to click my link, that's the giveaway.

WOULD YOU LIKE A SANDWICH?

Here's one of my favorite analogies: If you think about drinking more than you think about sandwiches, that's a red flag.

How often do most people typically think about sandwiches? Twice a week? Three or four times? Never? Every so often you may think, *I fancy a sandwich*—and you buy a sandwich. You eat your sandwich, and you enjoy it. Then the next day you might have a salad.

Later in the week you might have another sandwich or maybe not. A sandwich is something you enjoy from time to time but don't give much thought to.

When someone has an appropriate relationship with alcohol, they really don't give it any thought. Do you think about alcohol the same way I think about sandwiches? I didn't think so. Otherwise you never would have picked up this book.

This is a simple concept, but our society has moved the goalpost so far that we no longer recognize what normal drinking looks like. Alcohol is a product made by companies for profit. The more you drink, the more they profit. So, they have a strong incentive to fudge what an alcohol problem looks like. Like, we're talking some serious camouflaging. Which is why abusive drinking has been redefined as normal, and we have created a culture where alcohol is inserted into every imaginable circumstance.

ASKING THE WRONG QUESTIONS

When you question your drinking, you probably compare yourself to other people who drink more than you and have more apparent consequences. You feel reassured that you're "not that bad," and then you think no more about it until the next hangover. But that nagging little voice doesn't go away, does it? Deep down you know you shouldn't be drinking this much.

Most drinkers ask themselves the wrong questions. Instead of asking, *Is my drinking bad enough to stop?* we need to ask, *Does drinking make my life better? Is this good enough for me?* If you're a parent, add this question: *Would I want my children to drink the same way?*

I don't want to put you on a downer, but please stick with me because I can imagine what you are feeling right now. You probably have an uncomfortable feeling in the pit of your stomach—a feeling of dread and fear that maybe you'll have to quit drinking for good, and if so, your life will be over.

Keep reading, my friend, because I have some good news for you. Not only is your life most certainly *not* over, but you are also going to find out that everything you thought about sobriety is entirely wrong—a lie, in fact. The truth about sobriety will blow your mind. I am not exaggerating. Tell that ball of fear in your stomach right now that you are just going to be open to the possibility of discovering something new. You are not making any commitments or decisions right now. You can change your mind at any time. Does that feel a little better? Remember, you can stop reading this book and go back to how things were anytime you want. You are under no obligation. Alcohol is always going to be there.

As we start this journey I want to clarify the difference between being "sober" and being alcohol-free. Sobriety is for people who have come to the point where they have recognized that alcohol is causing problems in their life and they need to stop drinking. It is about working on the deeper emotional issues that led to and perpetuated alcohol becoming a problem. *Alcohol-free* is a new term that people use and tends to mean people who have recognized that it's just healthier not to drink alcohol and want to socialize without it. They also want to create space in their lives for personal development. I use both terms in this book. Regardless of which one you identify with, you will find lots to benefit you in this program—from understanding how our perception of alcohol and sobriety has been manipulated to practicing the five pillars of sobriety to enhance your own personal development.

APPROPRIATE VERSUS NECESSARY

I grew up in the UK and did years of self-destructive drinking there, but I've lived most of my adult life in the United States. Although there are differences in the British and American drinking cultures, the attitudes that Western cultures in general have toward alcohol are similar enough that we can discuss them together. These cultural attitudes have played a big part in how we have ended up here.

Alcohol is deliberately associated with as many positive experiences and celebrations as possible. Most people can't even imagine a birthday party, Christmas dinner, wedding, coworker socializing event, school reunion, or weekend without alcohol. I believe it's fair to argue that alcohol is appropriate in many of those situations, but there's an important distinction between *appropriate* use and *required* use. We can do all of those things sober without our joy or fun being in any way diminished.

But the distinction between optional and required has been almost completely lost. We now view a significant number of events as inconceivable without alcohol. We have been persuaded that without alcohol, none of those events can be tolerable, let alone fun. We believe we need alcohol to really enjoy them.

What bothers me most is the expansion of events and situations that alcohol is now being associated with. I've even recently seen yoga studios offering yoga and wine events—because a toxin-laden, dehydrating, central-nervous-system-depressing substance is exactly what you want with your yoga session.

But the one that perturbs me the most is alcohol and mother-hood. In particular, those cute little memes on social media and T-shirts that are meant to be hilarious. For example:

- "Kids happen. Wine helps." No, it doesn't. It makes you feel tired and cranky.
- "I'm the reason Mommy needs wine" (seen on a onesie). Mommy needs a nap and some support.
- "They whine. I wine." I get it; parenting is hard.

You can probably name half a dozen more. Please stand back while I exhaust myself with eye rolls. Okay, thanks, that's much better.

The "Mommy needs wine" drinking culture is screaming that being a mother is so grim that you need alcohol just to survive it. Men reading this book may be tempted to skip the parts about women's drinking, but this applies to you as well, as male culture also uses humor to reinforce abusive drinking habits.

What I take particular issue with is the dishonesty around drinking, especially binge drinking, which is deceitfully presented as fun and without consequences. There's a myth that there are only two camps of drinkers: those who can't handle it (full-blown alcoholics) and everyone else (the majority who can handle it just fine). In reality, *many* people drink to excess who don't fit the definition of an alcoholic, but they definitely face consequences—hangovers, embarrassment, depression, anxiety, spending too much money, loss of opportunities, or the dullness alcohol brings to your mind and soul. We use our spin-doctor skills to turn our consequences into a humorous story to entertain our friends, while burying our shame, embarrassment, and self-disgust.

We have normalized abnormal drinking by brushing away its severe and frequent consequences. It's a collective and deliberate denial that alcohol causes any consequences whatsoever to the vast majority who can "handle it." Hangovers are shrugged away as insignificant and irrelevant. Alcohol is fun, something we need; it is our right. And it is now being inserted into all parenting activities.

This new "Mommy needs wine" culture strikes me as a barely concealed primal scream. Women lack the support, childcare, and community that are necessary to raise a child. Being a mother is demanding, exhausting, and lonely. Which makes it easy to buy into the lie that alcohol is the best way to create the connection and relief mothers are craving.

Mothers are desperate to hold on to some part of their former selves because motherhood is way, way harder than they expected. And if they can't get proper support from their society or spouses, at least they deserve a drink! Women have, of course, been culturally conditioned for decades to believe there is nothing wrong with deserving or rewarding themselves with alcohol. Holly Whitaker describes this culture in her book *Quit Like a Woman*. She points out how alcohol marketing misleads women and deliberately obscures the devastating consequences to their health. She also emphasizes that research and paths to sobriety do not yet reflect women's unique needs.[1]

I believe the hypocrisy of the "Mommy needs wine" culture falls apart when you view how white women drinkers and women of color drinkers are perceived and treated differently. Cute memes and jokes about drunk mommies are seen as harmless fun when it's a middle-class white mom. But how would a mother of color be perceived? Would a drunk mom of color in charge of her kids be seen the same way? How would *she* be judged? Do you think that Child Protective Services would see this differently? The idea that "Mommy needs wine" is something that is unquestioned for middle- and upper-class white women. Women of color and working-class women would not be afforded the same luxury.[2] I asked Grachelle Sherburne, a licensed clinical social worker and psychotherapist what her thoughts were and she told me the following:

> The accepted notion that has been perpetuated in our society that mothers NEED to drink wine to "make it through" motherhood is an example of white privilege. If there was an organized group of women of color, socially drinking in a public place with their babies on their hips, the Department of Family and Children Services would be called immediately. As a social worker, I have seen calls being made to Child Protective Services on families of color, but for the same situation, resources, and support be given instead to white families.[3]

Doesn't that shift the perception of whether the "Mommy needs wine" drinking culture is harmless or not?

The companies that benefit from excessive drinking have quietly, cleverly, and very successfully inserted alcohol into places it doesn't belong, with no focus on the true costs of drinking. Contemporary mom culture is one of the most insidious examples.

WHAT ABOUT MEN?

Throughout their lives, men who abuse alcohol are treated very differently from women who do the same.[4] Drinking to excess is a significant part of male bonding, fraternity culture, sporting events, and almost every traditional major life achievement, from a graduation party to a wake. In the UK when a man becomes a father it is *expected* of him to get blind drunk. It's called "wetting the baby's head." However, the problems for men are also generally internal as well.

Not to reinforce stereotypes, but it's true that society in general still limits the emotions that men are allowed to feel. Anger, triumph, and apathy are fine; anything else is uncool or unmasculine. Alcohol, however, provides an acceptably masculine opportunity to unleash other emotions. Drunk men are given a free pass to weep on each other's shoulders or yell out "I love you man!" or lament the defeat of their favorite sports teams. They're allowed to express sadness about a job loss, a breakup, or a death in the family if they are drinking.

But without alcohol? A man who cries at the office after being fired would never hear the end of it. Neither would other kinds of emotional outbursts, like crying when you're sad about something, be accepted. Until society really and truly encourages men to express their full range of emotions while sober, the lure of excessive drinking will remain potent. For men, alcohol can be a powerful vehicle that finally allows them to express feelings, a reprieve from the restrictions that have been culturally imposed upon them. The construction of masculinity is very entwined with alcohol use and abuse of what it means to be a man.[5]

THE LAND OF FUN, EXCITEMENT, BELONGING, CONNECTION, RELAXATION, REWARDS, AND ROMANCE

At this point I hope you can see how alcohol inserts itself into as many places as possible as a solution to whatever problems we are struggling with. But the reason that alcohol is so insidious is because we have been convinced it's the best vehicle to get us to the land of fun, excitement, belonging, connection, relaxation, rewards, and romance, or simply, The Land. That's a long list, covering so many important things we all want and need as part of a satisfactory human experience. I mean, who *doesn't* want to go to that land? I know I did and still do. But it's not always easy; many of us feel like we don't fit in, that we are on the outside looking in. As we struggle to achieve those things, how tempting it is to reach for a quick, easy, inexpensive solution that requires little effort on our part. We just need a couple of drinks, and—abracadabra!—we are in The Land, *or at least perceive ourselves to be.*

We have absorbed this message so entirely that most of us believe at an intense level that giving up alcohol would mean being cut off from ever visiting this land again. A devastating thought! That's why drinkers tell me that quitting is the last thing they want to do—even when it's abundantly clear that alcohol is causing unpleasant consequences—and why they persist in their efforts to control or manage their drinking or to get back to drinking "normally," long after they have crossed the line.

It's not really giving up alcohol that's terrifying—it's the belief that we would be giving up our entrance ticket to that wonderful, mythical, elusive land. And this faulty belief is why you are struggling.

THE GOOD NEWS

Believe it or not, this is good news, and you're actually in a fabulous place right now. I know that feels hard to believe, but please trust me. You have no idea what will happen next, but I do. In the rest of this book, I'm going to prove that not only can you stop drinking and stay stopped, but you can also be happy being yourself, enjoy full connection with life and those around you, and never miss out on any fun.

I'm going to show you how to get to The Land without alcohol and—here's the kicker—why it's much, *much better* that way. I know that's a hard idea to absorb, because it contradicts nearly everything you've learned, heard, and seen since childhood. The truth has been deliberately concealed from you by the forces that want you to keep drinking.

I'm not asking you to take my word for it. At this point, all I ask is that you keep an open mind, as we explore a dramatic shift in how we perceive alcohol. I want this book to be a bridge between the two lands.

CHAPTER 2

The People Who Don't Want You to Get Sober

Before you take a leap of faith to stop drinking, there are a few things you need to do to prepare yourself. First, you must contact your doctor to ensure that you're quitting safely. Whether you're a daily drinker or not, the withdrawal effects from alcohol dependence can be harmful, even deadly. Alcohol dependence is when we are physically addicted to alcohol (typically drinking every day). But even if you're not alcohol dependent, please make sure you get appropriate medical advice before you stop.

But in terms of preparation, checking with a doctor will be the easy part. The hard part is getting ready to face the people who don't want you to get sober.

MIRRORS

We often surround ourselves with mirrors. We tend to consume alcohol with people who have a similar relationship to alcohol that we do. For many of us it's our families, the friends we grew up with or went to college with, or the people we work with.

There is an agreement among us that this is how we drink. It could be binge drinking on the weekends or happy hour after work. Group drinking reflects back to us that we are "normal" because we are all doing similar things. Drinking alcohol is *expected* of us.

I need to warn you that those people are *not* going to be happy you're giving up alcohol. You will make them anxious, because, generally speaking, as a culture we don't understand why anyone who didn't have an obvious problem would willingly stop drinking alcohol. In fact, most of my clients tell me that their friends would be shocked if they knew they were considering becoming alcohol-free. Because we judge how people are doing by what we can see on the "outside," if you are employed, have a home, go on vacation, and so on then how can alcohol disagree with you? But what my clients feel about themselves on the *inside* when they drink is the reason they want to stop. Even if you're only drinking a couple of glasses of wine but are finding you don't like the headache you get the next day or you ended up gossiping about a mutual friend and would really just prefer to socialize with a nonalcoholic beverage, you will still get pushback, because people who drink alcohol want the people around them to be drinking alcohol too.

If you've been drinking the same way they do, and now you've decided to stop, what does that say about them and their drinking? The last thing they want to consider is whether their alcohol consumption has a cost to it or is a problem. Drinkers only want to see alcohol as a benefit, and it will bother them that you are reflecting back to them that it has a cost as well. So, I need to prepare you for lots of pushback from other drinkers.

The first thing to remember is that when other people talk to you about your drinking (or your new sobriety) *they are not actually talking about you.* They are talking about themselves. They're trying to persuade themselves (by trying to persuade you) that their alcohol use is healthy, normal, and nothing to worry about.

These people—supposedly your caring friends, family, and colleagues—will appear in several different guises: the sudden addiction experts, the goalpost movers, the drunk persuaders, and the fun police.

The Sudden Addiction Experts

One common source you might get pushback on your sobriety from is someone who overnight became an expert in alcoholism/addiction (I know; amazing right?). These people will reassure you that you don't have a problem, because you're not like so-and-so who has a *demonstrable* drinking problem. Or they'll say, "It's not like you drink every day. You've gone days without drinking. You can control it. You're fine!" These reassuring sudden addiction "experts" will say that if you were like that other person (who really does have a problem), of course you should quit, but since you're not like that person, don't worry! They act as if they are well qualified to give you their "diagnosis."

Their real goal, of course, is to reassure themselves that *they* don't have a problem, by disproving yours. One of the ways they do this is by presenting benchmarks of people who are in much worse shape. For instance, as long as you are not homeless, throwing up all over yourself, passing out at work, or drinking straight vodka when you're home alone, then it's all good. It's so easy to Google a couple of facts and feel confident in telling others (usually unsolicited) that they can drink alcohol, as they do not have a problem. These supposed experts may also make "helpful" suggestions like taking a night or two off every so often or having a soda in between drinks. And they will be adamant that nothing you have said or done constitutes an alcohol problem, and you do not need to quit. Case closed! But beware when they tell you all is well and give you a reassuring pat on the shoulder. They do not have your best interests at heart.

The Goalpost Movers

These friends go even further than the sudden experts, by constantly and cleverly moving the goalposts of what defines problematic drinking. They have an opaque "line" between what is an alcohol problem and what isn't. In this way they can "fudge" what actually defines unacceptable drinking behavior, and they will make that line magically vanish whenever they feel like it. Thus, you can never actually cross the line and have a drinking problem—what a relief!

Expect to hear comments like "I know we said that if we ever got arrested, threw up on ourselves, fell over drunk in front of the kids, got a ticket for a DUI, or needed to skip work due to a hangover then that would mean we had a problem, but . . ." There's always a "but," and they will then give you a detailed rationale as to why those red flags don't actually count in your circumstances, and that you therefore haven't crossed the line. Maybe you were stressed or someone was mean to you or you got dumped or you were fired or it had been a tough week. Anyone would drink under those circumstances! You haven't actually crossed the line—not even close! Hurrah! Gin all 'round!

The Drunk Persuaders

These people are especially fun. They are inevitably quite drunk when it occurs to them that you've been nursing a Diet Coke all night. This makes them feel very sad since you are clearly missing out by not drinking. Being rather selfless folk, they take it upon themselves to persuade you to have a drink. They consider it their moral duty. They may corner you to get you alone and launch into a seemingly endless monologue about the pleasures of drinking. They can be quite urgent and insistent, but of course it's only because they care about you so deeply.

In reality, it hurts these drunk persuaders to see a sober person having a great time at a social event. As far as they're concerned, you're not simply making a choice, you're breaking a serious rule of the universe. They have to stop you from breaking that rule before you undermine their entire philosophy of alcohol.

As they continue their monologue, they will often repeat themselves, go off on tangents, and lose their thread. They may slur some words and have a little trouble keeping themselves steady. If drinking red wine, their lips will be stained, and they may even dribble slightly. What a charming example of the pleasures of excessive drinking.

The Fun Police

These people are deeply troubled that you have deliberately chosen a life devoid of fun. Their brows will be furrowed and their heads tilted as they try to process the mental arithmetic of having fun while sober. You can almost see the wheels turning inside their brains. But their programming since childhood is too strong to overcome. They simply won't believe that being sober doesn't have to be boring or joyless.

Although they may claim to understand and even applaud your attempt not to drink, they will also pity you for giving up every chance to have fun for the rest of your life. They will take it upon themselves as their sacred duty to urge you to "just have one" because it's Christmas, New Year's Eve, their birthday, your birthday, the weekend, a holiday, and so on. Your consistent rebuttals will pain and baffle them as they continue to try to make the sobriety math add up: head tilt, furrowed brow . . . nope, still can't get there.

HOW TO DEAL WITH PEOPLE WHO DON'T WANT YOU TO STOP DRINKING

You will invariably meet variations of all these characters when you first get sober, and they can all be dealt with in the same way. The following is a plan that will help you in your early days. Don't worry; this gets easier and easier over time, but at the start you may find this useful.

Strategy 1: Be Prepared. If you expect and prepare for this sort of pushback, you'll be more equipped to weather it. Always remember that your decision not to drink frightens drinkers. They don't want to change their own behavior, and they don't want you to make them look bad. You are mirroring something they don't want to see. So, their strategy is to get things back to how they were, with you drinking just as much as they do. Get ready to have your sobriety questioned and challenged, because they perceive your sobriety as a personal criticism, if not an existential threat.

Strategy 2: Have a Plan. When you are around friends and family, especially during a classic drinking situation, plan to arrive late and leave early. If possible, identify a safe person to hang out with, someone who isn't going to pressure you. Engage them in conversation and listen to them; this will take your mind off things. Look for opportunities to be helpful (clearing plates, getting chairs, and so on). Rehearse what you are going to say when you feel ready to leave. Keep it simple and polite and be firm. Expect pushback and just repeat that you had a lovely time, but you have to leave as you need to get up early. Don't stay longer than you want to stay.

Strategy 3: Don't Take the Bait. Do not accept *any* invitation to get into a discussion about your drinking. Those on a mission to persuade you to start drinking again will try to lure you into a debate, then push all your emotional buttons. The most effective way to resist these people is simply to listen without replying. Remember, they are not actually talking about your drinking; they are talking about their own. They are trying to persuade themselves. So, it's really important to know that this conversation isn't personal, it's not even about you, and definitely isn't worth your time to engage.

Practice listening to them without commenting beyond something harmless like "oh, that's interesting." Do not under any circumstances try to explain or justify why you aren't drinking, or you'll end up feeling resentful and persecuted. When they run out of steam, politely say, "Thanks for that," and walk away. This may drive them crazy, but that's not your concern. Your priority is standing firm in your decision and not having to defend it to anyone.

DO *NOT* TRY TO PERSUADE OTHER PEOPLE TO STOP DRINKING

While we're on the subject of peer pressure, please note that you should never try to persuade anyone else to stop drinking, and that includes your spouse or partner. It just simply won't work. I know it can be challenging to stop drinking in a home where someone else drinks, but it is possible.

Drinkers are still tied to the belief that alcohol benefits them. If you try to change their minds, they will interpret it as asking them never to visit The Land again, and they will be horrified and disgusted. There are no words to persuade them otherwise until they reach a point when they're ready to see sobriety as a good thing for themselves.

Until then, the most powerful way to demonstrate the awesomeness of sobriety is simply to go about your business of being sober. When you stop drinking and follow the program in the chapters ahead, your life will transform. You will look better, your relationships will improve, you will get more done, unexpected opportunities will come your way, and you'll have just as much fun if not more. Others will notice, including your former drinking buddies. And that will be a more powerful message than anything you could say to them.

CHAPTER 3

Crossing the Bridge into Sobriety

Stopping drinking is not just about stopping drinking.

You may have already discovered that. You have probably made more than one attempt. I know it can be frustrating and exhausting. You set a date, get prepared, and put your best foot forward. Things go well at the beginning; you can't believe how much better you feel, and you have a spring in your step. Then out of nowhere, with no resistance, you have a drink and another, and you are drinking more than you want to again. Nothing has changed; you discover that when you wake up that sense of shame and self-loathing quickly makes an appearance. You are back to square one.

Damn it.

Please don't despair. This is not something that can be achieved with willpower. In fact willpower is pretty useless when it comes to quitting drinking. This is because alcohol is not your root problem. Yes, you read that correctly. Alcohol, as mentioned earlier, is a symptom of your problem but not the underlying problem. Let me explain. An alcohol problem is a combination of our subconscious thoughts, childhood wounds, environment, and inability to deal with difficult feelings and emotions. We use alcohol because it's an effective and powerful way to run away from or numb all of this stuff inside of us that we don't know how to deal with. It is these factors that create an alcohol problem.

When we start our drinking careers, it's usually "fun." It's new and exciting, the bridge to adulthood. There is always a cost, even if it's just a hangover (but what's a hangover when you're seventeen, right?); however, we perceive that the benefits far outweigh that cost. Some of this is true and some of it is perception. Falling over blind drunk when you're nineteen can be spun into a fun tale of debauchery; less so when you're forty-nine. When we look back, we may be surprised to see that the little gremlins of shame, self-disgust, fear, and self-loathing made appearances in our drinking careers much earlier than we realized. If we couldn't rationalize them away, then we developed little coping strategies: food, consumerism/shopping, screens, and spinning tales about our behavior so it all came out in the wash.

But those uncomfortable, unpleasant feelings don't just vanish because we want them to. They linger in us, and because they are uncomfortable, we push them into a storage container deep inside of us and seal the lid real tight. These feelings accumulate and fester inside of us.

Let's just be honest here; adulting is hard. We're not prepared for all the things we have to learn to deal with as an adult: our first broken heart, career disappointment, friendship groups shifting, and so on. Then there is the harder stuff that so many of us have gone through, like abuse and trauma. We don't seem to live in a world that really prioritizes our emotional well-being. Instead it prioritizes what is outside of us, what we have, achieve, get, look like, and so forth. We don't have the language to speak about our feelings or the skills to manage our mental health, so we just soldier on using outside sources to fix inside problems.

Let's look at the math here. We have feelings that are difficult to manage, and we have a readily available, cheap substance that is promoted and encouraged in just about every aspect of our lives that magically numbs all those unpleasant feelings away. Even better than that, it creates a temporary feeling of euphoria and promises to take us to The Land, all for about twenty bucks!

Who could resist that deal?

Do you see the problem? It's not the alcohol. Because when you stop drinking you have a storage container inside of you filled with feelings and emotions you have not dealt with, combined with a mindset that is undermining you and often sabotaging you. When we use alcohol to take the edge off of how we feel or to fit in or be liked, then we sacrifice a little bit of our authenticity. And it is the erosion of this part of us that causes pain. And that is why you drink more than you want to.

Are you now thinking, *Oh, crap! I thought she was just going to tell me there was a magic switch or something? I want to stop drinking, not rake over my past.*

Because yeah, I get it. But this is not bad news; nor is it as hard as you think. In fact it is easier. Drinking when you don't want to is hard. Sorting yourself out so you no longer desire alcohol is much easier.

We need to change what is going on inside of us; it's basically an inside job. And that's where we have to start.

When I was drinking, I probably came across as a happy-go-lucky party girl. I was always up for the party, always wanted to be in the center of the action, as that is where I believed The Land was. I was fairly unreliable and inconsistent. I messed up quite a lot, but I muddled through life somehow. If you looked at me you would probably think I was doing "okay." I had some of the outside stuff—a job, home, college degree. But what you saw on the outside was completely at odds with what was going on inside. Inside, I felt lost and broken, and despite always being in the center of the action, I was filled with loneliness and despair. The more I tried to connect with people, the further away they seemed; sometimes I managed it, but it was fleeting, then gone. I was full of "wanting" but nothing ever satisfied me. I moved houses, jobs, and countries, each time believing that the change would fix me. I moved from relationship to relationship, thinking the right man would save me. I thought I was following the instructions to get to The Land, but whenever I thought I was there I realized I wasn't. But I persisted. I kept up a pretense that everything was fine, but inside I just wanted to die.

I didn't really want to die. I just didn't know how to live. I also didn't know that "not drinking" could be a thing. And I had no idea what my real problem was.

The answer lies in quitting booze and transforming your internal experience. So eventually your insides and outsides match. That's how you get to The Land.

THE BRIDGE

If you can go with the metaphor of travel for a little longer, then I want to let you know that to get from the land of alcohol to the land of sobriety you have to cross "the bridge."

There is no other way of getting to The Land except by going over the bridge, and the length of the bridge is different for everyone. But I can tell you how it feels, and you are going to need to know this in advance, as preparation is everything and is the key to your success. So, here are the things to know about the bridge: it's weird, it's uncomfortable, and other people won't get it. This is just the experience of being on the bridge. The reason for this is that as you journey across it, you are going to experience a shift in mindset. Mindset is the framework in which we see, experience, and process the world. It's how we make sense of it: Me + drinking = fun. Me – drinking = boring.

This is the mindset of alcohol use. Alcohol is fun, so I have to drink to have fun and for people to *perceive* me as fun. It is this mindset that keeps us stuck in the conundrum of drinking when it's really time to stop. We are aware of the consequences. We don't like them, but we believe that we *need* alcohol to have a fulfilling, normal life. So, we think that's just how it is.

But it's not.

This is an ingrained and deeply rooted mindset. Do not underestimate how much you have bought into it and shaped your behavior around it. It won't shift overnight. It's a process (I use that word a lot) that will shift as you continue over the bridge.

I also want to prepare you for how you will feel when you first step onto the bridge. It's usually a mixture of fear, hope, excitement, shame, and a lot of grief. Because alcohol is such a big part of everything, don't underestimate how uncomfortable the early days of not drinking will feel. It may take several attempts. Please don't look on that as failure. It's not. I see sobriety as a seesaw. On one end is sobriety and on the other is drinking, and we just need to put enough weight on the sober end so that it eventually tips down and embeds itself. The more information you have and the more help you have, the easier your experience will be. If this was a problem you could solve by yourself, you would have already done so.

THE FEAR OF MISSING OUT

Over and over, this fear of missing out, or FOMO, is the main reason people hesitate to quit alcohol. Despite overwhelming evidence to the contrary, they still perceive alcohol as benefiting them and bringing them something that without alcohol they could no longer get.

This is by far the biggest misconception that drinkers have. Marketing and reinforcement from our culture and peer groups tell this story over and over. As we have seen, the alcohol industry is in business to make a profit. It makes money by persuading us to buy more of its product, which it does by convincing us that its product will give us feelings and experiences we covet and desire and give them to us quickly. It's simple math: Alcohol = fun, excitement, belonging, connection, relaxation, rewards, and romance. No alcohol = none of the above. Can you see how if you believed this, quitting alcohol would feel like the worst thing ever?

And it is this belief that makes quitting drinking feel so hard. But it doesn't need to be. It only requires a simple shift in perception. But to get that shift you first have to understand the con. What you have been persuaded to believe about alcohol isn't true. Alcohol doesn't deliver on its promises.

Eventually, some become so battered and beaten that they glumly accept with great reluctance that they need to stop drinking and that their life will now be boring and dull. I know how they feel because I was one of them. I was twenty-seven when I stopped drinking. It seemed like members of my entire peer group were still going out to pubs and clubs and having a wonderful time. And here I was resigning myself to becoming a hermit.

I was willing to do this because alcohol had brought me such chaos and destruction. I was so unhappy and uncomfortable in my own skin that I was willing to do anything just to get some peace and safety. I had completely given up on entrance to The Land. I felt sure that my life was going to be gray and boring, that I would never go out again, never dance, and certainly never get laid again. I would be an outsider, and I was resigned to this because I just couldn't live inside myself anymore.

I need to let you know that much to my amazement, my life did not close down when I stopped drinking; it expanded—from black and white to Technicolor, with bells, whistles, and marching bands added on. (Well, the last thing isn't true, but you get what I mean.)

It was then that I realized how much I had been lied to by alcohol advertising and by the culture I grew up in. Combine this with an inability to deal with my emotions and feelings and suddenly I was the perfect candidate for an alcohol problem.

Now, I want to say that I have no quarrel with people who consume alcohol. Many people can take it or leave it. Some of us can't. My problem lies in the dishonesty around our relationship with alcohol and that no one ever talks about how high the cost of drinking is for too many of us. This is where the problem lies.

THE COST-BENEFIT ANALYSIS OF ALCOHOL USE

If we all looked at how much alcohol costs us, then our relationship with it might change. Just to be clear here, I am not talking about money. Although, it is an interesting exercise to add up how much money you spend on alcohol. Not just the money you spend on buying it but also cab fares, take-out food, lost items, missed opportunities, and so on. I think you will find the total a real eye-opener. The other aspect to consider is how much time does your relationship with alcohol take up? How many hours a week do you spend drinking and recovering from drinking? We can always make more money, but we can never get time back.

But the cost I am really talking about is the unseen price we pay: the embarrassment of how we may have behaved, the shame we may feel at something we did or said, the casual sex we may have had that feels deeply uncomfortable the morning after, the broken relationships, the little bit of dignity we lost when we fell over and everyone laughed at us, or the dangerous situations we can encounter when intoxicated, not to mention the effect it has on our bodies and our minds. Alcohol is a depressant, and if you drink regularly you are going to start feeling depressed because that's just science. There is also the cost to our integrity when we become someone we don't recognize, someone we wouldn't want our children or our parents to see, as well as the cost to the people who have to clean up after us—our families, our coworkers, our children. All of these things add up to a price we pay every time we abuse alcohol.

What's your cost? Ask yourself, *Is it worth it?* Because in all honesty, if you look at how much alcohol costs you and if you feel the price is worth it, then all I can say is carry on and good luck! I would like to tax you further to pay for the extra policing and health-care costs incurred by your abusive drinking, but honestly, apart from that, I have no objections.

But I do believe that if everyone who abused alcohol on a regular basis had a true look at what it really costs them, they would be horrified. And if you peer a little closer, the whole idea that it's fun begins to fall apart a little bit too. Have you ever wrapped your arms around your "new best friend" on the next bar stool only to avoid them in the grocery store the next week, with a feeling of shame flooding your body and no idea why? Have you ever had a rousing time drunk with a bunch of people and felt that alcohol helped you bond deeply, only to discover that they were fair-weather friends who had no idea of who you really were?

The biggest price I see people pay is in their precious bandwidth. Alcohol costs us scope and breadth. It costs us energy, resources, and time, and we have to decide if our relationship with alcohol is worth that loss. Going through life without full access to this bandwidth is like having to put up with 2G internet. I mean, it works, but the video and downloads are slow, and pictures don't load. It's frustrating that we can do *some* things, but not everything the way we want. But for some reason we put up with it because it hasn't occurred to us yet that we don't have to drink, that we could actually live our entire lives not drinking and be completely fulfilled and happy, with access to 100 percent of our bandwidth.

We only have finite resources, and I'm going to hazard a guess that the average drinker loses about 20 percent of their bandwidth to alcohol. When we still have that 80 percent, we have our jobs/careers, we can go to college, pay our rent, and have a holiday or two. We can do all the outside stuff, so everything looks the way it should. But what we can't do is fully grow into the people we are capable of being. Things are a little fuzzy, and we would like to give this a little bit more thought because it feels important, but for some reason, we just don't have the . . . yep, you guessed it, bandwidth!

You know what I'm talking about right? Drinking, thinking about drinking, thinking about *not* drinking, recovering from drinking. These things take up time, energy, and space in our heads. When you look at the cost-benefit analysis, you can see that alcohol is not worth the price you pay. Imagine who you would be or what you could do with that magic 20 percent back. The reason that extra 20 percent is magic is because that is where our growth is. It's where our extraordinariness is. We will discuss this later in the pillar of growth, but it's important to understand now that if we want to grow into the people we are capable of being, we need that missing 20 percent.

Lastly, I just want to say that I know lots of people can use alcohol safely and mostly harmlessly. I have several friends who use alcohol in this manner; it's not the main event but in the right circumstances, it can add a little spark to an evening. These people, however, do not depend on alcohol to have fun or feel like they belong. They already feel like that anyway. Alcohol is just something they use from time to time. They may have a sore head in the morning on occasion and that may have motivated them to drink less often. However, more and more people are recognizing that even a sore head is too much of a cost and want to experience what an alcohol-free life could be like. Wherever you are on your journey you will find much here to support you in your alcohol-free life.

THE GRIEF OF LETTING GO

Let's examine grief for a moment. Grief is an emotion we feel when we lose something or someone we care about or let go of something or something ends. The grief process of denial, bargaining, anger, sadness, and acceptance has been well-documented, and we will go through these feelings when we let go of alcohol, because for so long alcohol was something that we believed we loved. And although that sounds crazy, because alcohol is basically just a substance with no thoughts or feelings of its own, what we loved about it is the perception that it took us to The Land. Perception is a tricky thing because it may have taken us there once, or it may have taken us there many times, but if you are reading this book now, I know it hasn't taken you there in a while. Just think on that for a second: When was the last time alcohol kept its promises to you?

Alcohol sometimes feels like our best friend. It is always there for us, it never lets us down, and it provides us with a few minutes of exquisite release. And letting go of all of that, the promise of alcohol, is going to feel sad. That's normal and it will pass, and you will undoubtedly look back and laugh at ever feeling that way.

But it's not just the grief of saying goodbye to alcohol that you will experience; it's also the grief of letting go of the identity you have constructed as someone who drinks.

Releasing this identity of who you thought you were is part of the process of grief and letting go. I identified strongly with my party girl image (the reality was completely different), and in my head I liked the images of me looking sophisticated while drinking cocktails.

And alongside this loss of identity we also have the faulty belief that sobriety is going to be glum, boring, and dull. So not only do we have this image of ourselves as a party girl, sophisticated wine drinker, beer lover, whatever. We also have the question of who we will be without alcohol. Is our new identity forever going to be a boring person sitting at social events looking grim and nursing a glass of water?

At this point all you can do is trust me. I know you are probably a bit suspicious, because like most people, you are going to need to see evidence of what I am telling you, and you've got none. All you have is the absence (or the thought of absence) of alcohol and the devastating feeling that goes with it. You have lost something you care about, and the grief process is kicking in. You feel bad, and no one wants to feel that way.

I'm going to suggest that the best way to get through the grief process is to accept and acknowledge how you feel. This is really the first step in beginning to respond to your feelings differently. Don't try to suppress or deny it. Tell someone (who understands) how you feel and get busy with getting across the bridge. These feelings will pass, I promise you.

So, what do you do now?

You are in a really great place right now. I am not patronizing you. You are on the brink of change—in fact, you are on the brink of life-expanding change. That is not something to be taken lightly; it is huge. I feel very excited for you, because I know what's in store. You are about to start on the journey of becoming the person you were meant to be. Enjoy the ride. If you are serious about this and want some extra accountability, then take action. Send me an email—I'm totally serious—with the subject line "I'm done with alcohol" and tell me why you want to commit to living alcohol-free. If you are ready to take this plunge then I am here for you. Email me at veronicavalli@soberful.com, and let's get started.

PART TWO

Building an Alcohol-Free
Life That Works

CHAPTER 4

The Five Pillars of Sustainable Sobriety

In my years of living sober and two decades of experience working with clients, I have discovered that there are five pillars to sustainable sobriety. By "sustainable sobriety" I mean sobriety that requires no effort, no willpower. It just *is*, and you just *are*. And it feels great. In fact, sobriety is so attractive to you that you just want more of it and all that it brings. *Imagine that.*

Everything worth having is worth working for. Creating a sober life will take some effort, energy, and focus. Everything you put into it you will get back in abundance. That's why I invite you to join the program—your program—by implementing the five pillars below:

1. Movement
2. Connection
3. Balance
4. Process
5. Growth

We will be going into each of these pillars much more deeply in subsequent chapters, but before we do, I would like to provide some background on them. Bear with me; this is important.

First, you may be asking, *Why do I need a program to stop drinking?* This is not an unreasonable question. Put most simply, the pillars of the program are there to support you. They are the edifice around which you rebuild.

As I have already mentioned, willpower will not get you sober. In fact, willpower won't get you very far at all. Willpower works a little bit like a muscle: eventually it becomes fatigued, so when you need it most, you won't have the strength to resist drinking.[1] Plus, willpower takes effort; it feels exhausting. We want sobriety to feel easy, natural, and effortless. It's not that getting sober doesn't take effort, it does, particularly at the beginning, but it's how we apply that effort and energy that is key to the outcome we get. It takes a lot of effort to spin your wheels and not actually get anywhere.

The fact that you are reading this book shows that you have recognized that it's not simply a matter of stopping drinking or even willpower. To quit alcohol successfully we have to get to the root of the problem and embark on the deeper inner work. Some of that inner work is the messaging we have absorbed that alcohol is the only way to have fun or relax, and that will take a little while to undo. Whether we are getting drunk most nights or just feeling pressured into attending after-work happy hours, we are drinking because of how we think it will make us feel.

We are going to learn a new language, a new way of being. We are going to shift our mindset, and we are going to develop emotional literacy. Our *feelings are the engine of our behavior* and this is why we have to do the deeper work. We all have feelings. We have hard feelings, uncomfortable feelings, and painful feelings as well as wonderful feelings. Of course, we would all love to be joyous every single minute of every day, but we can't be. We were all born with the potential to feel the full spectrum of our emotions, and they all serve a purpose. We simply can't know love without knowing loss and sadness.

The problem is not that we have to experience difficult feelings and emotions sometimes; it's that we don't know how to deal with them when we do. So, we try shortcuts such as numbing them, running from them, or just pushing them down deep inside us. You've probably done this yourself. I know I did. I grew up in a family of origin that finds big feelings unacceptable, and it was implicitly communicated to me that my big feelings were not acceptable. So, as a young child I learned to push them down inside of me. When I was disappointed by something or hurt or frustrated, I just pushed those feelings into my storage container. This felt really uncomfortable, but I had no other guidance or role models to show me it could be any other way.

Before I even picked up alcohol, I was using behaviors and food as a means of dealing with these uncomfortable feelings. I would binge on sugary snacks, I would binge-watch TV, and I smoked cigarettes (the true gateway drug). And then I found alcohol. This not only allowed me to quickly and effectively numb my feelings, it also had the added bonus of making me feel comfortable in my own skin for a few short hours. Alcohol was a good thing in my life. It made good things happen, and I loved the way it made me feel. So, my relationship with alcohol from the get-go was about how it made me feel. I was predisposed to its power because as a teenager I needed something to help me with the maelstrom of feelings inside of me. And bingo! There it was.

So, when we stop drinking, and we no longer have this golden substance to numb us, what are we left with? Yes, you guessed it—lots and lots of feelings. The early days of not drinking can often feel like an emotional roller coaster. It can feel really weird living in a world where alcohol use is everywhere, but we are abstaining from it. We will have to navigate life a little differently. Plus all of those feelings that have been in our storage container for years begin spilling out all over the place. I often hear from clients that they have no way of knowing how they are going to feel from one moment to the next and that their feelings are unmanageable. Because of this, it is enormously helpful to have support from people who know what you are going through and a clear plan for how to deal with everything you are feeling.

Because misusing alcohol prevents us from growing, and we have all these feelings to deal with, we need a personal development program to help us through. We need instructions on how to live our lives to get the results we want. Assuming that how we have been living previously is unsatisfactory, we need to find a new way, and this is what a program is—a method of personal development for sober people.

Using a program to live your best life is not about ceding your autonomy to someone or something else. A program is something that makes you a better you. There are several models of recovery already out there. There are, of course, the twelve steps of Alcoholics Anonymous, the SMART Recovery model based on rational emotive behavioral therapy, Refuge Recovery based on Buddhist principles, and Women for Sobriety based on the thirteen acceptance statements, among others.

All of these programs, including Soberful, exist because we need a framework to deal with our feelings and to grow as human beings in ways that we just couldn't when we were younger, and when we were drinking. Very simply, a program is a road map into the life you have always wanted but never thought possible.

Incidentally, these five pillars are not just for people with an alcohol-use disorder; they are personal development principals that will facilitate growth, change, and transformation in anyone who is seeking it. Also, their application is not a one-shot deal. It's not like you do them and then you're done. They provide structure and momentum for the rest of your life. They are there to support, help, and guide you, because as humans we are ever growing and changing. Our circumstances will never stay the same, and we have to meet these challenges. Life in many ways is one long lesson we have to learn, and we never graduate from life. Life will patiently wait for us to learn the lesson we need to learn so that we can get to the next experience. If we don't take the opportunity to learn, then the lesson will just come around again and again.

GROWTH: FEELINGS AND EMOTIONS

Before we get started I want to explain the difference between feelings and emotions. They seem to be the same but are also, confusingly, different, and it's worth noting the difference. Emotions are hardwired into us and are an intrinsic part of human behavior.[2] Recent research has suggested we have only four basic emotions—happiness, sadness, anger, fear[3]—but this is still often debated. Emotions feel very immediate and are connected to our body's survival system. We experience our emotions physically as a sensation in our bodies. Fear is the easiest one to understand in this way. In the earlier days of human evolution, we needed fear to tell us when to run from the animal that was trying to eat us.[4] Fear is an internal, physical, and immediate emotional experience. We can't ignore it, and we have to respond to it.

Feelings are then provoked by our emotional events, and we experience them consciously in our minds and thoughts first. Feelings are subjective and filtered through our own personal experience.[5]

So, I might feel fear that I was going to get fired from my job. I would feel the emotion of fear as a physical sensation (my heart would race and so forth) because my perceived safety is being threatened. Then I would experience feelings in relation to this emotional experience. These feelings could be those of guilt (I've let my family down) or shame (I'm not good enough) or something else. The way I experience *feelings* related to the *fear* of getting fired will be personal and based on my own history. The feelings of guilt and shame would come from beliefs I hold about myself, and the event of getting fired would feed into these beliefs. Feelings are what make emotions personal.

SUSTAINABLE SOBRIETY

I want to say a bit more about why sustainable sobriety is important. I've already mentioned that willpower won't help us to get sober because, like a muscle, it is a finite resource. So, once it gets depleted you have no defense against the desire to drink when this desire is triggered. And it will be triggered. Triggers to drink alcohol are everywhere. We may feel determined one day never to drink again, but when we are triggered by external conditions or internal feelings, our willpower is useless. Using willpower to stop drinking just feels like you are trying to swim against the current: eventually you will become too tired to fight and the current will win.

Sustainable sobriety, on the other hand, is sobriety you don't have to think about. It just takes care of itself when we focus on the five pillars. And once we accept that we are walking away from alcohol for our benefit and not missing out by doing so, we take away alcohol's power over us. The reason it feels hard at the beginning is because we don't know how to live sober. A lot of our alcohol use is played out on autopilot. We drink because everyone else does. So learning to live sober is really like learning any new skill: at the beginning it feels hard, it's unfamiliar, and like we are not getting anywhere, but if we persist then we will get more competent, things will feel more natural, and we will eventually become masters. Quitting drinking will help us learn emotional mastery and feel fully connected to ourselves. When we feel fully connected with all parts of ourselves then the only things we want to do are things that are enriching, rewarding, and fully aligned with who we really are.

At this point, you may be tempted to ask, *Does that mean I can drink socially again one day?* And the answer is that it's unlikely. And here's why. As I have mentioned before, we are very enmeshed in a cultural belief system in which alcohol is considered only as a benefit. This messaging is powerful and comes from many different angles. For example, how many TV shows do you watch where the characters drink alcohol? Nearly all of them, right? And unless those characters are acting out a specific addiction story line, the alcohol consumption typically looks glamourous, sophisticated, and fun. But how often do you see the consequences?

There is a TV show on Netflix called *Dead to Me* that my husband and I usually enjoy. There was an episode early in the second season where the two main characters were upset and emotional and were up late drinking wine in bed. (Lots of messaging there that it's okay to use alcohol to deal with difficult feelings.) The clock showed 12:30 a.m. and they were still talking, so they probably didn't get to sleep until say, 2:00 a.m. The next scene was the morning after. It was a school day and the mom was cooking breakfast for her kids, so it must have been around 7:00 a.m., possibly earlier. She was fully made up, her hair was blown out, and she looked fabulous, no sign or mention of a hangover or only having about three or four hours of sleep.

Who does that in real life? The true consequences of drinking alcohol until 2:00 a.m. on a weekday were not shown. If this was portrayed accurately, the kids would be burning Pop-Tarts in the toaster, while the mom had her head down the toilet. It was a complete misrepresentation of alcohol use. But we absorb the messaging of the big glass of red wine, and we think we will have the same experience as the one we are witnessing on the screen. But we don't, as that image is a lie. This is really powerful and misleading messaging, and it's all around us.

The reason quitting feels so hard is because of our belief system around alcohol, and I have been calling on you to really question those beliefs. As long as we feel it is the best way to get to The Land, we are always going to feel like we are missing out if we give it up. But when we develop a serious alcohol problem and are eventually forced into quitting, we can sometimes still harbor the notion that one day we can drink the same way that we enjoy a sandwich, the way we see everyone else doing (again, perception not reality). The desire to drink *normally* (I use that term loosely) is based on how alcohol is represented to us (benefits with no consequences). What we want is *that*. We want to be like the women or men we see on TV or in ads who have a beautiful glass of wine and experience no consequences. So wherever you are in this journey, if you start drinking again you will more than likely continue drinking the way you did before you stopped—with the same consequences. And nothing will have changed. You wouldn't have picked up this book if you were happy with that, and the whole point of this program is to find a way to have all the things we want without alcohol.

ALCOHOL DEPENDENCY AND SOCIAL DRINKING

Certainly, lots of people try to manage their relationship with alcohol and drink *socially* without consequences. And typically they find it takes a lot of effort. First, there is the term *social drinking*, which is very ill-defined. It means different things for different people. To a large extent in Western culture, we have also normalized abnormal drinking. So, what is seen as "social drinking" is actually abuse. But because so many people do it—and have a car and a house and a job—they can rationalize that they don't have a drinking problem. Our belief system tends to be that someone who has a drinking problem drinks 'round the clock then passes out. As long as you are not *that*, you are fine. So, the term *social drinking* is really meaningless. We will bend it to mean what suits us.

But more challenging than this is that alcohol dependency (physical and psychological) can lead to neurobiological changes in our brain. We don't need to be physically addicted to alcohol to experience these side effects.[6] Our brain chemistry will be working against us. This also shows up in our tolerance to alcohol. How you drank ten or twenty years ago is not how you drink today. The reason for this is that your body has had to learn to tolerate alcohol. It adapts, and we don't feel the effects of alcohol like we used to, which is why we need to drink more to get the same effect. Research is also showing that along with impacting our brain chemistry, our habitual use has also impacted the reward-related neural processes in our brains.[7] It's like when we start drinking again after a period of abstinence. Our brains remember how much of this substance is required to get the buzz we are searching for, and we are back where we started.

So to sum up, is it possible to become a "social" drinker (insert your own definition of what this means) after abusing alcohol? I don't think the answer is yes or no, but when you do a cost-benefit analysis and understand what alcohol use costs you and learn that it is changing your brain chemistry and damaging your health, why would you want to try? It takes a huge effort, and for what? Why is alcohol that important and necessary to you that you are willing to invest all this energy into moderating your consumption? Does it not strike you as ludicrous? I repeat: the only reason you want to try is because of the internalized belief that alcohol brings you something you can't get anywhere else, and that just isn't true.

If you are feeling a little despondent about this, don't be. Remember that there is another way to get to The Land. You won't be missing out on anything. You will be gaining, and even though you may find that hard to believe because you can't see it yet, it's true. You may also be thinking that maybe some of this doesn't apply to you, that you're "not that bad." Because you are reading this, I'm going to say that your relationship with alcohol is troubling you. Actually, let's reverse that and ask the question again: Are you living the life you want to be living? It's not about how bad your alcohol use is, it's about whether your life right now is good enough for you. Are you prepared to settle for the way it is? Is this how you want to feel? How you want things to be till the end of your days?

Again, no one ends up here by accident. You are seeking something. You want answers, you want change, and the five pillars of sustainable sobriety are how you get it. The five pillars all work together—they not only help you hold up your sobriety, they are tools for life. You don't just use them for a bit and then leave them in a cupboard. Alcohol was your crutch, and the pillars are going to replace that crutch with real tools for personal development, so you can make your existence here mean something. With the five pillars you will have an instruction manual for managing your feelings and emotions and dealing with the ups and downs of life. As a consequence of this, your life will expand in ways that right now you can't even imagine.

The need and desire to drink will subside. Sometimes it takes a few weeks or months, and it can come in waves, but it will go. Alcohol will begin to fade into the background, and you won't really notice it. You will have become someone who *doesn't drink*. Not someone who can't, won't, shouldn't, or is afraid to drink. Think about that. When you get to that stage you will have moved from not being able to think of a reason not to have a drink to not being able to think of a reason to have one. This is the fact of the matter.

I am now going to take you across the bridge from the land of alcohol to the land of sobriety. The way to get across the bridge is to learn how the five pillars work and how to apply them to your life. In each pillar description I have added journal prompts—questions to ask yourself that will help you get deeper into understanding the pillars.

Remember, you are *not* alone on this journey. All over the world there are millions of people waking up and deciding they don't want to drink anymore and are finding a more fulfilling way of living. You could be one of them. Let me be your guide across the bridge.

CHAPTER 5

The Pillar of Movement

There are two levels to the pillar of movement. Simply put, the first level is that we need to move our bodies. Movement is one of the best ways we have to take care of not only our *physical health*, but our *mental* and *emotional* health too.

There is another layer to movement, and that is being *purposeful* about the *direction* of our lives. Misusing alcohol can throw us off course. It takes up a lot of time and energy that we could be using on things that really matter to us. We lose connection to ourselves and our purpose, and we don't move in a direction that is right for us. What are you moving toward? This pillar is about reclaiming ourselves and using exercise to manage our mental and emotional health.

MOVEMENT: PHYSICAL, MENTAL, AND EMOTIONAL HEALTH

When I started researching this part of the book, I thought I was going to write a simple outline of why exercise is good for our mental health because of the dopamine hit we get when we move our bodies.

Sometimes the answer we have been looking for is staring us in the face. It feels like stating the obvious to write a chapter on why exercise is good for you. I do, however, believe it needs to be said. Sometimes the solution is much simpler than we imagine it to be. Sometimes, there really is a magic bullet that can solve multiple problems for free or for very little money—and that magic is movement.

I didn't think I wanted to say much more than that, maybe quote a few pieces of research. Then I discovered Kelly McGonigal's book *The Joy of Movement*,[1] and it opened up a whole new level of understanding of why movement is not just the foundation of our human experience but also of our sobriety. I realized on a much deeper level why movement was so essential to our well-being. It seems that the dopamine kick[2] we get from moving our bodies is just scratching the surface of the benefits of exercise. What the research reveals is that the complex chemicals the brain and body release when we exercise are purposefully designed not just to lift our mood, but to help us feel less lonely and more connected, sleep better, have less pain, and develop a sense of love and connection toward our fellow humans.

That's pretty much all the things that most of us use alcohol for. It's not a straight swap. Putting down the drink and just exercising every day isn't quite enough—we also need what the other four pillars bring to our lives. But you can already see why exercise needs to be a substantial part of an alcohol-free life.

Exercise to Heal Our Brains

We know that alcohol and drug use interferes with our brain chemistry. Interestingly, the effects of alcohol on the brain are more complex and less understood than the effects of drugs. As Judith Grisel puts it in her book *Never Enough*, "Alcohol is a neurological sledgehammer."[3] That means it affects nearly all aspects of our neural functioning.

Understanding how our brains have been affected by alcohol at a very basic level can be helpful as we navigate our path into sobriety. It is this chemical interference that can continue into early sobriety. Grisel outlines how regular drinkers will see a "down regulation of endorphin synthesis,"[4] which feels like a case of the blues. We will feel low and uninspired and that life is just gray. Some people can shake off that feeling in a few days, while others use alcohol and other substances to try to lift their mood, creating a dysfunctional cycle of using alcohol to deal with the consequences of alcohol.

I used to drink from Thursday evening through Sunday. Monday through Thursday were pretty blah. I would feel low, hungover, unproductive—life just felt like a trudge. Thursday was usually my best day. My body and mind had more or less recovered from the previous weekend, so I wanted to drink Thursday evening. Drinking would give me a buzz and everything felt great. Friday I would be hungover, but the thought of drinking that evening would keep me going until Monday morning, when my body just couldn't take it anymore.

We drink on the *promise* of alcohol rather than the reality of what it delivers. As we have discovered, there is a gaping hole between the two. When we feel low, of course we want to feel better. Our brains will selectively ignore our last few experiences of alcohol and give in to the misleading promise that this time alcohol will improve everything. This is because when we first drink alcohol it makes us feel good and relaxed, and we focus on these initial effects and forget the consequences.

As we explored earlier in this book, much of this is because of the misguided belief about how alcohol benefits us. We have been programmed to believe it helps us, makes us feel better, and improves our lives. All of those beliefs are held subconsciously and have been presented to us via external sources, such as marketing, culture, and peer groups, which is why a lot of our behavior is on autopilot.

The conscious mind asks, *How can I feel better?* and the subconscious mind replies, *Alcohol!* So, we often feel we are drinking without really having made the choice to do so, and this is why process work (as explained later in chapter 8) is so important. Process work helps us understand why we do the things we do. Otherwise we are just working against ourselves. You can see how it becomes a cycle. Human beings can't tolerate feeling low for an extended period of time. We naturally don't like discomfort and want to fix it. If we believe alcohol is a solution, we will keep turning to it for answers.

We ingest alcohol to make us feel better and depending on our circumstances and brain chemistry, we may feel euphoria and fleeting relief. But rather than truly uplifting us, alcohol works as a central nervous system depressant.[5] It will actually contribute to depressive feelings[6] and lead to a sense of general malaise, which ironically is the exact opposite of the feelings we were initially seeking with our alcohol use.

When we drink and use drugs, we interfere with the brain's ability to create the chemicals it needs in order to feel good. This is why exercise is so key for an alcohol-free life, and why it offers so much more than a quick dopamine kick. The chemical response we trigger when we exercise actually begins to *heal* our brains.[7]

Our brains' reward system is very ancient and was designed to keep us alive by rewarding us for the behaviors that benefited our survival. Exercise will trigger the reward chemicals we need to feel good, and it will reduce cravings and increase the receptor sites we need in our brain for the feel-good chemicals to dock in.

The more receptor sites, the more we get the benefits from the feel-good chemicals.[8]

But that isn't all. We were made to move. Our bodies and our brains were designed to get us moving and keep us moving. Whatever type of movement we engage in, there are opportunities to connect with other people and become part of a group. Movement that involves other people also increases our sense of connection and belonging. And as McGonigal emphasizes all through her book, creating joy in movement is one of the best experiences we can have.

When I take on a new client, exercise is one of my nonnegotiables (safely detoxing from alcohol is the other). They need to commit to some form of movement on a regular basis. If someone is starting from the couch and the idea of exercise feels completely overwhelming, we begin with very small goals.

To get started, we look for how the client can incorporate walking into their daily schedule, with the goal being to walk at least five times a week for a minimum of thirty minutes. To make this fun and attractive, I ask them to put a playlist together of all their favorite music or to download podcasts or audiobooks. I frequently use exercise to double up on other things I need to do. I get through a lot of nonfiction books while I'm exercising. If I'm able to absorb information while I'm exercising, I can make this a double win.

Moving needs to become part of our routine. We just do it no matter what, and the more enjoyable it is, the easier it will become. Now, I'm going to confess that regular exercise is a constant challenge for me. I am no athlete. I can't run fast, I'm not strong, and I don't want to win anything. I just like how it makes me feel. Over the years I've done lots of different things from circuit training to yoga, swimming, bike riding, and running. But exercise changed for me after I had kids. I went from being someone who moved every single day in some shape or form to someone who went weeks without properly exercising.

Becoming a parent is a shock to the system. Nothing prepares you for the exhaustion. When my kids were very young, I just muddled through. My only chance for exercise was a gym that had childcare. On a good week I could get there maybe three times a week—which never felt like enough.

When we first had kids, we only had one car, as my husband would bike to work. One day the car had to be serviced, and to make it easier I said I could just walk my son to day care in the stroller. It was about a thirty-minute walk, and after dropping him off, I went to my office. I walked in and just felt amazing. At that time, I wasn't feeling low or depressed—I was in a pretty good place even if I was still exhausted a lot. When I sat down at my desk, I realized that the reason I felt amazing was that I had just walked for about an hour. The contrast hit me quite hard—like I said, I hadn't observed feeling down or low, but just an hour's walk made me feel like a million bucks. I wanted to feel like that every day, and I realized that I was overthinking the exercise part and making it too hard on myself. I was trying to exercise the way I did before I had kids, and it just wasn't working.

My belief was that I needed to work out for at least an hour for it to be worthwhile. If I was going to get hot and sweaty then it needed to be for a decent amount of time. I really didn't think anything less than sixty minutes was worth it. I was wrong about that. I was actually choosing to do nothing rather than do less than an hour of hard-core exercise.

Now my attitude has completely changed. If I can exercise for an hour, then that's a big victory, but now I'll take whatever I can get. My window to exercise is really in the morning—I want to get it done before I do my hair and makeup, as I do a lot of video calls for my business. So sometimes that means getting up early to work out before my kids wake up or trying to squeeze something in later in the day.

I still only get to the gym about three times a week, but in between that I'll do an intensive thirty-minute exercise video at home or, if I'm really stretched, I'll just walk laps around my park when my kids are playing. Bingo! I had found another way to just keep moving, to get that endorphin kick and feel like I had done something positive for my mind and body. All I needed was to shift my perspective. I would truly love to work out hard every day, but the circumstances of my life—by which I mean kids and sleep needs—just don't permit it that often. But if I can do something physical every day, I can get those feel-good chemicals flowing.

The point of telling you all this is that you may find yourself in an exercise rut and have a lot of really good reasons why you can't do it right now. I want you to know I've been there. It's important to separate the idea of movement from the idea of fitness. Fitness is great—we want to be as fit as possible—but the purpose of this pillar is to experience the chemical reaction only movement can provide. Look at your schedule, look at where you can squeeze in some more walking, and make it a must. If something feels like a "must," then it is more likely to happen.

Even with kids and a busy schedule, there is some time when you can fit in a thirty-minute walk. If your challenge is time, like so many of us, take a hard look at where you spend your time and see what you can change. Don't set yourself up to fail; start with ten minutes if that's all you can manage and go from there.

When we carve out this time we are also saying, *I'm worth this*. You are worth this; your well-being is worth this. We are doing this because we value ourselves.

For those of you who never let your drinking interfere with your workouts, you are about to discover how amazing those early gym visits feel when you are not hungover or dehydrated. I can't tell you how many clients I've had who drank most nights and were still hitting the gym the next morning at 5:30 a.m. and powering through. It was almost like a badge of honor. Who cares if they drank a few glasses of wine by themselves the night before if they were still up with the larks and pounding the treadmill?

What actually happened is that they had just become used to exercising that way. The exercise helped lift their mood that the alcohol had sunk. Feeling hungover and powering through anyway just felt normal. Living that way isn't sustainable no matter what your constitution. At some point it sneaks up on you and makes everything harder. After a couple of months of sobriety, many of my clients report feeling transformed. They were working out without feeling tired and dehydrated. Bringing movement into our lives is an act of self-care that we all need.

Exercise as an Addiction

I want to mention that although I wholeheartedly think exercise is a wonderful thing, we never want to let it get out of balance. Don't let exercise become the new fix. Don't obsess. Balance, balance, balance. I want to be clear here that there is a difference between exercise as a healthy habit and exercise as an addiction. Behavioral addictions, like exercise and gambling for instance, meet the same criteria as chemical addictions, such as tolerance, withdrawal, loss of control, unintended consequences, and so forth.[9] I wanted to bring this to your attention: if we have had a previous addiction, we are more susceptible to transferring that addictive behavior to something else.

If we totally rely on exercise and the feel-good chemicals to help us manage our mental health without doing any of the other necessary work, we'll find ourselves in trouble, because there is always going to be a time when we can't exercise. We either get injured or circumstances prevent it, and we begin to see our mood crash really quickly.

If movement is our only strategy for managing our mental health, we will start to struggle really quickly when we can't do it. It bugs the hell out of me when I hurt my back and can't exercise for a couple of weeks. I feel it. I don't feel low exactly—it's more just a mild frustration. But my first workout after an enforced period of nonmovement always feels amazing.

My point is that if the only pillar you are working on is movement, there will be a time when you can't move and your mood will crash. We need to do the deeper work of sobriety so that we have other tools to manage our mental health. There is a careful balance that needs to be maintained here. We should never exercise in a way that compromises our family's needs, our employment, or our physical health. We mustn't push our bodies so hard that we injure ourselves. Instead, we need to adjust to our changing circumstances and conditions and balance how and when we move. It's a priority that we need to consciously pursue to balance our well-being.

Journal Prompts to Get Our Bodies Moving

If you already move and exercise, is everything in balance? Or are you exercising too much at the cost of other needs?
  Example: *I tend to be all or nothing.*

If you are not exercising, what feels possible for you right now? Can you take a fifteen- to thirty-minute walk?
  Example: *I would like to. I think I could walk during my lunch hour for fifteen minutes.*

How can you create more space and time in your day to move?

Example: *I can walk instead of scrolling on my phone.*

How do you feel when you exercise?

Example: *I feel great.*

...

MOVEMENT: PURPOSEFUL DIRECTION

The second level of movement is figuring out what we are moving toward and being conscious about the direction we want our lives to go in. What are you moving toward or away from?

When we drink more than we want to, we sacrifice our authenticity. When we are having a couple of glasses of wine to fit in or getting drunk and embarrassing ourselves, we are not being true to who we really are. We are moving away from ourselves by degrees. We may not notice this drift, as it is often quite subtle. When we stop drinking, we are given the opportunity to appraise how far we have drifted from our purpose and consciously move toward what is authentic for us.

At this point we have two choices: we can carry on ignoring the parts of our lives that aren't working and just drift, not going where we want to go, or we can stare them right in the eye, pick up the reins, and steer our life in the right direction.

There's really only one choice.

There are no excuses here. It is not too late, you are not too old, and too much has not happened. There is no better place to start than where you are right now. The future is unwritten. You can either be the author of your own script or an extra in someone else's.

Moving Forward One Square at a Time

Change happens by degrees, and we have to start where we are. We are not going straight to square one hundred; we are just looking for square one and then the next one after that and then the next. This is how we move toward our purpose. One square at a time.

Once we accept that we are at square one, we can look for square two. Now, it's hard to see where square one hundred is, and even if we can see it, it feels like there are too many squares in between. Remember no one gets anywhere without going to square one first.

We first have to accept and own exactly where we are, whether we like it or not (and often we don't). When we work the five pillars and start getting out of our own way, then we become more true to ourselves and more aligned with who we are and what our purpose is. We will discuss this more in the chapter on growth, but for right now we are going to start exploring how to move in the direction we need to be going in.

When I was drinking, I really didn't have any goals or purpose. I thought I was living life to the fullest, but all I was really doing was repeating the same mistakes in different places. I wasn't going anywhere; I was in a holding pattern. It was like being a little boat tossed around on the ocean with no rudder. I just drifted wherever the wind blew me.

There are, of course, many circumstances in our lives that we have no control over. It is a waste of our energy even trying to change them. What we do have control over is how we choose to respond to our circumstances. This is not to diminish suffering or trauma from circumstances beyond our control. On the contrary, we need to accept and validate what we have been through. I have had too many clients just dismiss or ignore massively significant events from their past. They just push them into the storage container. What happened to us *matters*, and we choose our response to these circumstances by first validating the fact that we have suffered due to circumstances beyond our control and that our feelings resulting from this are important. It's only by choosing to accept our feelings that we can begin the process of healing and change.

Understanding that this is how we move forward is key to an alcohol-free life. This is where all the pillars come together. Through process work, we begin to understand our emotions and feelings—instead of just reacting to them, we can observe them and choose our response. When we become attuned to our emotional life, we can heed the call to grow, and we can move toward that growth through aligned action. Aligned action is when our values, decisions, and actions all match.

Our relationship to alcohol is fueled by the way we believe it's going to make us feel. The choices we make and the actions we take are all influenced by how we think we are going to feel and a desire to move away from feelings that are unpleasant or uncomfortable. When we live this way we are not aligned with our values. This is how we become the little boat tossed around on the ocean. We can't use our rudder because we are just trying to survive the waves and not capsize. We can't go anywhere because we are just trying to get through day by day without going under. When we get sober, we don't have to live that way anymore. We can ride the waves, we can steer ourselves into calmer waters, and we can find a safe harbor.

To start moving in the direction we want to go in, we first need to be still and go inward to find balance—we have to pause and reconnect. Paradoxically, this kind of stillness is movement because it's purposeful. The purposeful pause can awaken us to where we really want to move toward next. Sometimes we use busyness and action as a strategy to not feel our feelings. If we are always "doing," we can kid ourselves into believing we are being productive, but we are really just distracting ourselves through misaligned action. We want to move purposefully while balancing all our needs. The pillars do not work alone to hold up our sobriety; they work together.

This is not about setting goals and checking them off or achieving things or even getting difficult things done. It's about *aligned purpose*. It's about what you were put on Earth to do. I was speaking to a client the other day who is qualified as an interfaith minister, and her calling is to help people with end-of-life services. However, she is not fulfilling this purpose because her alcohol use is getting in the way. My job is to get her sober, so she can bring her gift to the world. My aligned purpose is to return people to themselves by getting them sober so they can in turn fulfill their purpose. I want you to move toward your purpose whatever that may be. This work is not limited to people who want to quit alcohol. Everyone would benefit from evaluating what they want to move toward and what they want to move away from. This is an invitation for you to do just that.

The great thing about sobriety is that you will be able to achieve a lot and get stuff done. With all that extra bandwidth and *time*, you will be able to do things you can't even imagine at the moment. But this is a messy process. We often have to do a lot of different things to figure out what we *don't* want. It is a discovery process, and we often make a lot of mistakes along the way.

I was never one of those kids who knew what they wanted to be when they grew up. I had friends who wanted to be doctors or hairdressers or teachers. I had absolutely no clue. I wasn't good at planning and rarely set goals because I always knew I would fail to reach them, so I didn't bother. I was driven by how I wanted to *feel*. I wanted to be included, I wanted to belong, I wanted to feel happy and successful, I wanted to feel like I was in the thick of things and was significant. The actions I took were all driven by these feelings I was chasing.

Moving to London, traveling in America, going to college, choosing the men I dated—all of those actions were driven by how I imagined I would feel as a result. I believed life was a series of boxes to check. Partner, check. Buy a house, check, Have a career, check. Lose ten pounds, check. If I checked as many as I could then it would result in me feeling happy, content, and safe. I thought that was the deal (the secret to happiness). I thought external accomplishments would result in positive internal feelings. But I could never capture the feelings I was chasing, and if I did they were fleeting. Before I could even register them, I was back to frantically checking boxes, thinking this time would be different. If you look around you will see many people have fallen into this way of thinking. Whether they have an alcohol problem or not, they have gotten lost in the external world of box checking.

As a result, my behavior was very erratic. I would passionately pursue something and get all lit up thinking this was the solution (to everything) and that when I got this thing then I would feel amazing. Then I would abruptly reverse course when I saw something else I thought I wanted. I was always chasing. I thought I wanted the things I was chasing (the job, the house, the person), but what I was driven by was a belief that if I had those things, I would feel safe and finally be happy.

Needing to feel safe was undeniably the biggest motivator for me. A little boat on the ocean is not safe. I did not feel safe. I never really felt safe. I don't mean that I felt like I was going to be harmed or threatened; it was more like a feeling of quicksand underneath my feet. I didn't feel anchored. Subconsciously I was always looking for the thing that would assure me I was safe now, that I would be okay. But no matter how many boxes I checked, the ground never felt firm beneath my feet. So I turned to alcohol to calm my internal storm.

We can live our whole lives feeling this way. Always chasing, never arriving. Checking boxes, but never actually becoming what we are capable of being. I was working under the impression that I needed to arrange my "outsides" in order for my "insides" to feel okay. I was trying to address an internal problem with an external fix, and it just doesn't work that way. If I wanted to feel safe, whole, and connected, it had to come from within. This is the work of the five pillars.

When we stop drinking, we use the five pillars to uncover what is within us. We find out what it is we truly seek and why. We discover what our purpose is in the world. I know for a fact that your purpose is not drinking when you don't want to because you are scared other people won't think you're fun, drinking so much alcohol that you feel sick, obsessing over alcohol, regretting drinking alcohol, or wasting energy trying to manage alcohol. That is not your purpose; it is a distraction. You haven't found or fulfilled your purpose because managing your complicated relationship with alcohol has taken bandwidth and energy.

Purposeful movement is a process of peeling back the layers of hurt, limiting beliefs, and "shoulds" so that we can discover the direction we are being called in. We are not going to achieve this on day two of our sobriety. It is the work of our lifetime.

I went to college, I had jobs, I moved around a lot (and I mean *a lot*, as I've lived in about forty different places), and I was still without any direction in my life. I could plan the weekend, but I had no idea what I wanted to achieve in life, where I was going, or where I would end up. I just hoped it would all work out without me having to actually do anything about it.

Sobriety gave me the ability to change that. I did not, on day one of my sobriety, think that someday I would write a book that helps other people get sober, or that I would want to be a therapist and create an online platform. All I knew on day one was that I didn't want to hurt anymore. When I stopped drinking and getting in my own way, I became more purposeful.

Getting sober gave me a career. I took an addictions-counseling course and loved it. From there I became a psychotherapist. I had always been intrigued by what made people tick. I just never realized there was a job actually based on that. I absolutely love the realness of psychotherapy—being allowed into someone's internal world has always been humbling and fascinating for me. The realness and vulnerability of it awes me every time.

Each time I moved to the next square and felt comfortable, the next move would open up—not just in my career but in all areas of my life. It happened in my personal development, in my relationships, and in my ability as a mother.

Things unfolded in different ways. I made mistakes. I took jobs that were based on my ego rather than my abilities. Relationships didn't work out. All of that is par for the course—it's how I learned. Helping people get sober and becoming a speaker and advocate for sobriety is what I want to do in the world. I had no idea that a fascination with what made people tick, along with my alcohol problem, would lead to this. But here I am, and I am right where I need to be. I want this for you too—your version of it. I want your path to unfold, and I want you to *let it*. There is a you-shaped hole in the world and only you can fill it.

Acceptance: Letting Go of Struggle and Getting Unstuck

When I think about my life when I was drinking, it always felt like a struggle. I'm not talking about when I was drunk but all the times in between. Everything felt like a struggle, from getting through the day with a hangover to just getting the stuff done that needed to happen, like paying bills or applying for a job. Nothing flowed.

It's true that there are many worthwhile things we can do that take tremendous effort and feel like a struggle, and the investment of energy is worth it. But what happens when we are lost in the details of our life is that we end up struggling against ourselves. Letting go of the struggle is about accepting where we are so we can move forward.

Acceptance is a form of surrender—it's surrendering the struggle. It's letting go of outcomes (tough, I know), and it is letting go of control (even tougher). In truth, we have very little control over our external environment. I'm writing this book in the middle of lockdown during the COVID-19 pandemic. Like millions of people all over the world, my external world has changed dramatically, and I have no control over when this situation will end. All I can do is accept that this is happening and choose how to respond.

Now, I don't have to like what is happening, and often we won't. Pushing, resisting, and struggling are not going to change the reality of what is. Those actions will just deplete our energy. We will have lots of feelings about the external event, and we want to feel those so we can process them, learn from them, and release them. Then we have to accept what is, where we are. This is where I am. This is square one. We may not like it, and we don't have to like it. But accepting the reality will help us see square two.

Struggling and pushing against our reality will just keep us stuck. The need to struggle in this way comes from our belief that if we control our external world, then we will get what we desire and feel the way we want to. Accepting what is doesn't mean we have to like it or that it doesn't need to change. We don't have to accept the unacceptable. Instead, we accept where we are, and we take action to move in the direction we want to go.

Take a guess at what your purpose is. There is no perfect answer. Just write the first thing that comes up that feels true. It can be vague or laser-focused. These prompts are about cutting through the minor details so that we can see more clearly. Listen to the voice inside. What are your feelings trying to tell you?

Example: *To be a good parent, to play music, to help others.*

What does square one look like for you? Remember, we may not like square one, we just have to accept this is where we are for now.

Example: *See a therapist, join a sober program, tell my partner I'm struggling with alcohol, accept that I don't want to drink.*

...

Getting Clear on Our Purpose

Purposeful movement is really an unfolding. That's why I've used the analogy of a board game. We just have to start and then see what unfolds. It is a cliché to say it's the journey and not the destination, but very few of us can move toward our purpose and have everything work out just the way we want. The lessons are in the unfolding and how we choose to respond.

It is through those experiences that we learn the lessons we need in order to go to the next square. In fact, we can't get to the next square unless we have made mistakes. Those mistakes and messes are what equip us to go forward.

In order to stay true to our purpose, it helps to understand what we value. When we understand our values—what matters to us—we can move forward with purpose. This is where process work comes in. Many of us have drifted away from our values during our relationship with alcohol. We have behaved in ways that are not aligned with our values, but just the opposite. This will cause us to have feelings of guilt, shame, and remorse. That is why healing and restitution is required.

Remember, we can't change our past, but we can choose how we respond now and in the future. Getting reconnected with our values is part of the healing process. Values are usually fairly stable; they don't fluctuate a lot, but they may evolve as we grow and change.

Getting clear on your values will help you enormously with purposeful movement. It will help you make decisions and take action based on your values. You will be able to identify what is for you and what is not for you.

Purposeful Direction: Assessing and Reasserting Our Values

When I did this exercise I saw that I was completely out of alignment with my core values. Integrity and growth are two of my core values, and I couldn't have been further away from them if I tried. When I saw this clearly I felt them burn inside of me. I wanted to live a life aligned to my values of integrity, growth, connection, love, and joy. And this meant I had to make changes in my life. This is purposeful movement.

To discover your values so you know what you are moving toward, try the following:

1. Brainstorm your core values. Some examples include well-being, health, kindness, success, honesty, service, safety, independence, fun, belonging, justice, strength,

freedom, friendships, stability, trust, curiosity, growth, passion, balance, power, wisdom, integrity, spirituality, joy, gratitude, challenge, risk-taking, peace, and ambition. You can also search online for additional lists of values, such as the one in "Live Your Core Values: 10-Minute Exercise to Increase Your Success" on taproot.com.[10] Spend some time exploring these and write down four or five that really stand out for you.

2. When you think of these values, what feelings do you get? Do you get an inner pull? Do they matter to you? If so, why? Why are these values so important to you?

3. Would you be comfortable with other people knowing that these are your core values?

4. How can you live with these values? What actions do you need to take based on these values? How can you move toward them?

When we get clear on our core values, our actions will become more purposeful, and the direction we are going in will be aligned with what matters to us. Now, the direction may feel challenging: when we uncover these truths about ourselves, we may have to make some changes. We may find that we are doing things that are not aligned with our values, and this is a lot of the reason why we struggle and feel uncomfortable in our own skins. We feel uncomfortable when we are not behaving in ways that are true to who we are.

Sobriety gives us the opportunity to become who we really are by living our values. Please understand that this doesn't mean being perfect. We will all take actions that are not borne of integrity. We are only human. I have made choices (usually out of fear) that went against my values and lived to regret them. I have had to make restitution and learn painful lessons. This doesn't make me a bad person; it makes me human. I want to live my values to the best of my ability and forgive myself and learn from the mistakes so that I can do better next time.

MOVEMENT AS A PRACTICE

To recap, we are going to practice moving in two ways. We are going to move our bodies purposefully, regularly, and joyfully. When we do this we make a commitment to our well-being on every level. Physical movement is the cornerstone to your sobriety. If you are looking for a place to start, this is it.

Second, by using the journaling prompts and exercises in this chapter you are bringing your awareness to the direction you want your life to go in—what you are moving toward and what you are moving away from.

Becoming purposeful about the direction we are moving in and taking action aligned with our values is how we reclaim ourselves in sobriety. Putting down the drink is the first square. Reclaiming ourselves through inner work is what makes our sobriety rich, fulfilling, and sustainable. We drink because of how we feel. When we act in ways that are out of alignment with our values, we feel bad, and when we feel bad for long enough, what happens? Our minds search for relief. We will go deeper into this work when we explore the pillar of growth because sobriety and movement will inevitably lead to growth.

When you begin the process of reclaiming yourself through the movement pillar, you are taking out the best insurance for never drinking again. You are creating a foundation for your sobriety to stand firmly on.

What are you moving away from?

> Example: *I want to move away from the drinking culture; I hate it. There are certain people that I know aren't good for me and there are behaviors (like gossiping) that I want to stop because I know that's not who I really am.*

How does it feel to not know what the next square is?

> Example: *Scary, I want to run, but I also don't want to go back.*

Do you want what you want because of how you think it is going to make you feel?

> Example: *Yes! I am always chasing things and people because of how I think they are going to make me feel. When I get that, do this, become this, then I will be happy, safe, fulfilled. But whenever I get what I want, it doesn't feel the way I expected.*

What would you do if you weren't afraid?

> Example: *The thought terrifies me, but there is so much I've always wanted to do and be but fear has always stopped me. I would _____.*

What are your five core values?

> Example: *Love, loyalty, joy, success, and well-being.*

...

CHAPTER 6

The Pillar of Connection

Connection is our lifeblood, and the need for it is universal—none of us can get by without it. Money can't buy it, you can't order it on your phone, and you can't fake it. Authentic, real connection is something we recognize deep in our souls.

Connection is as essential to human beings as air, food, and water. Without it we suffer and fail to thrive. When we are tiny babies, we need connection to our primary caregivers. We understand this as secure attachment. We know that without that strong physical and emotional connection babies cannot thrive, and children cannot reach their potential.

As Laura Markham says in her book *Peaceful Parent, Happy Kids*, "When children feel securely connected to us, they learn to love themselves and to love others. The old saying that we give our kids roots so they can later grow wings is as true as ever, and as ever it requires a secure bond for those roots to really sink in."[1]

As we grow, our need for connection evolves; it never goes away. As we are all unique individuals, our need for connection with others will vary greatly, but it is still a very important need that must be met. Alcohol is presented in our culture as a quick, easy, and effective way to achieve connection. But is the connection we achieve when drinking deep and meaningful enough to nourish our souls?

When we drink too much, we don't always make the best decisions—we say and do things we regret and cause hurt, confusion, and sometimes chaos, and these things can't always be brushed off the next day. We can't be consistent and solid in the way our relationships need us to be. If we are having a couple of drinks to "fit in," we are not showing up as our authentic selves, and our connections are not as meaningful as they could be.

When we are full of shame and regret or just hungover, it interferes with our ability to connect. As we continue to behave this way, our shame increases and our self-esteem decreases. Shame and low self-worth become obstacles to the meaningful connections we need to thrive. When these feelings grow, we begin to dislike ourselves, and we don't want people to get close and see these unlikeable parts. The problem then becomes more compounded.

There is nothing worse than feeling disconnected from yourself—existing in the world but being completely disconnected from who you really are. This separation occurs when we begin to feel more and more uncomfortable in our own skin, and when this feeling creeps in, it needs a buffer. It's too painful to tolerate otherwise. If we use alcohol to act as this buffer, we lose ourselves just a little bit and then a bit more. When we get sober, we have to return to ourselves first for connection to be meaningful.

BELONGING TO YOURSELF

The path to belonging to yourself is via self-acceptance, forgiveness, and compassion. It's also about being authentic. You are the home you live in. I can't emphasize this enough. But this is a process that takes a little time and effort, and we will go into some of the work that is required when we get to the last two pillars. A dysfunctional relationship with alcohol stems from the abandonment of ourselves to meet our connection needs. Two of the most important needs we have are connection and authenticity, and sometimes we compromise our authenticity to be liked, approved of, and included. When we do this we feel uncomfortable within ourselves. And alcohol provides an anesthetic.

The journey of sobriety is really the journey of returning to ourselves. The most important thing is that you like yourself and that you *behave* in ways that enable you to like yourself. Because we can't belong anywhere until we belong to ourselves.

The first step to belonging to yourself again and reconnecting with who you really are is to stop drinking. Do whatever is necessary to make that happen. Then treat yourself with kindness and compassion. Give yourself time and space to rebuild your life, your self-esteem, and your self-worth. Begin to take small actions that feel honest and true to you. You are building self-awareness, taking time to pause and reflect and get curious about why you feel a certain way. It is not about being perfect; it is about being present in the human experience you are having and making that experience as authentic and true as you possibly can. Belonging to yourself is about congruence. This just means making your insides and your outsides match, so you can show up in the world as you really are and not how you think the world wants you to be. When you belong to yourself, you don't want to run away from yourself anymore, and that is the best feeling in the world.

USING SOBRIETY RATHER THAN ALCOHOL TO CONNECT

For a lot of people, the promise of connection and belonging is one of the primary motivations for drinking alcohol. It was certainly mine. I thought alcohol was the key to everything I wanted. As previously discussed, marketing and cultural representations of alcohol portray connection and belonging as a major benefit of alcohol use. This is very powerful programming and one of the major components of FOMO that people experience when they try to stop drinking. If alcohol tells you that drinking will lead to connection and belonging, then what is the opposite of that? That sobriety equals being alone and lonely? Who wants that? No wonder the *idea* of sobriety isn't attractive.

But the representation is based on a faulty belief. It is this belief in our subconscious that drives us to continue drinking, and for some, long after we recognize it's a problem. We labor on, believing that it will work if we can just get the components right—the right amount of alcohol at the right time in the right setting will result in our achieving all the things alcohol promises. You may have failed tonight, but there's always tomorrow. If you keep trying, surely you will one day achieve the holy grail of drinking alcohol while achieving connection, belonging, and fun with no consequences or embarrassment or hangover. It just takes effort, right?

If you have been trying really hard to get alcohol to deliver on all its promises, how often has it worked? And what was the cost? Is the cost worth what you received?

We can keep laboring under that belief system, or we can try another way. Sobriety is not just about the absence of alcohol, it is about connection, belonging, fun, excitement, and an expansive life. Without alcohol, there is more space to let all these things in. The incredible news is that you don't have to give anything up to get sober (apart from alcohol of course!). You don't lose; you only gain. It is our perception that is at fault, not the reality. We have been persuaded by marketing and our culture to believe things about alcohol that are not always true.

▶ Journal Prompts to Understand Connection

Have you used alcohol to feel connected to others?
> Example: *Yes, I have often gone for after-work drinks on a Friday because otherwise I would be on my own.*

What happened?
> Example: *I think years ago it felt like fun, but recently I've been drunk and then regretted it the next day and felt ashamed.*

Have you ever felt connected when alcohol wasn't involved?
> Example: *I used to be part of a community group. We would sometimes fall into these really interesting conversations that helped me understand people better. I would then feel closer to them.*

...

LONELINESS AND CONNECTION

Vivek Murthy, MD, explores loneliness and connection in his book *Together: The Healing Power of Human Connection in a Sometimes Lonely World*. He cites research that "identified three 'dimensions' of loneliness to reflect the particular type of relationships that are missing."[2] These are *intimate* or emotional, *relational* or social, and *collective* or community.

Intimate relationship needs include the longing to be really seen and known, the desire for closeness, and the validation that you matter and are loved. To sustain an intimate relationship we have to be vulnerable. Relational need is the desire for sustaining friendships or for groups where you feel like you belong and can contribute and where people would notice your absence. Collective relationship needs are about feeling part of a community or network.

Because loneliness can be broken down into these three areas, we can see it is possible to have a fulfilling intimate relationship and still feel lonely, or to have several close friendships but feel the loneliness from the lack of an intimate relationship.

I have had times in my life where I have had none, one, or two of these levels of connection and certain times when I've had all three. My constant relocation (as I mentioned, I move a lot—it just seems to be in my DNA) has sometimes made it hard to maintain all three, but I have been very aware of needing them.

In my early thirties I had wonderful and wide friendship groups. I had close friendships with my sober friends and best friends from when I was at college. After years of feeling like I didn't belong, I had several groups in which I felt a keen sense of belonging. I also felt like I was part of a community of colleagues. But while I was happy and fulfilled, I also noticed the absence of a romantic partner. *Where is he?* I used to think. Then I met my husband, and all three levels of connection were satisfied. But then we moved to America, and the other two levels fell away. I was very lonely for friendships, and I really missed having a best friend who lived nearby.

Many of us have to consciously notice which dimension of loneliness we are suffering from. Modern living can sometimes make this challenging, and moving to different areas, work demands, and technology can all make us lonelier.

I truly took my friendships for granted when I moved to the US with my new husband. I didn't expect to be lonely in the way that I was. My marriage was loving and supportive, and my husband is great company—we like doing pretty much everything together. However, I'm also a woman who loves having girlfriends. I like the camaraderie and the feeling of having a confidante to share the experience of womanhood with.

No matter what stage of life we are in, there are different types of loneliness that can impact our well-being. Alcohol is the devil that makes us believe we can bridge the gaps in our loneliness. It has inserted itself into so many of our social situations where it doesn't belong. Kids' birthday parties, yoga studios, cinemas—the messaging is that alcohol will make these experiences better. This is just market expansion: if you associate alcohol with as many things as possible, then there will be more demand for your product and increased profit. This is how we have normalized abnormal drinking. Thus alcohol and connection have become completely inseparable.

Being Lonely

We have an epidemic of loneliness in this world. So many of the ties that bind us are breaking, leaving us feeling disconnected. I don't feel we are creating a world that connects us more; I feel we are creating a world that separates us and reduces our "connection" to shouting at each other on social media.

Loneliness should be a public health issue. We now have substantial research that proves how detrimental it is to our physical health.[3] Loneliness costs us money in health and social care, and it is very much one of the driving forces behind addiction. The pain of loneliness is intolerable; it is one of the worst experiences of my life. It literally feels like death. Who can tolerate that? No wonder we drink.

Can you count the times you drank to feel less lonely? To feel like you belonged? Did you drink so you could be with other people? I know I did, and what I received back was a hollowed-out version of what connection can really be.

Loneliness is not solitude or the state of being alone. We can feel lonely in others' company if we feel disconnected. Or we can have connection in some dimensions, but not all.

I was very lonely when I was drinking. I never felt like I fit in or I belonged anywhere. I was with people a lot. I was always part of a group, but the connections I made never seemed to go deep enough or last long enough. The loneliness was the hardest part of my drinking. It's like an ache deep inside that you feel extremely ashamed of. I wanted to hide, as having someone witness my loneliness would be the worst thing imaginable, but of course this feeling just led to me isolating even more.

Feeling lonely feels like a defect of character. We feel like it is our fault that we are lonely—that there is something wrong with us. When we start believing this, it feeds our negative self-talk. This then leads to feelings of shame, and the shame compounds the loneliness.

When we feel shame, we don't want other people to see us; we want to hide. We don't feel worthy of being around other people. We desperately need connection or just a kind word, but we build walls around ourselves that keep others away. The pain of loneliness can feel unbearable, and it is easy for the alcohol to feel like our best friend.

One of the hardest things about living through the COVID-19 pandemic was how it forced us into isolation from one another. Enforced loneliness has taken its toll on our mental health, and we have had to work harder and be more creative about the ways we get together. We have had to work harder to maintain our connections, but despite the effort, connection is always worth it.

Square One: Acknowledging Our Loneliness

The first step to changing our loneliness is to recognize what we are experiencing. This is just being at square one. We can't make it better until we acknowledge the problem first.

I had a period of intense loneliness after I gave birth to my first child. I had just moved to a new place, and I had no support system, no friends, no family, and a new baby who didn't sleep well, so I was exhausted, which compounded everything.

I was having trouble breastfeeding and was referred to a lactation nurse. Her name was Theresa, and she was lovely. She made me feel safe and taken care of. I was going to see her three times a week with my son. I would look forward to those thirty-minute visits so much—they were the highlights of my week. She would listen to me, and I would really feel seen. She just had that mothering vibe that I really needed at the time. I felt incredible sadness when I realized I didn't have any more reasons to visit and then I realized that I was lonely. I was the mum who was taking my eight-week-old baby to every playgroup I could possibly find. I went to all of them desperately looking for connection. Eventually I found a group of mothers around my age that I felt a connection with. It changed everything for me. I got close to a mother who had a son the same age as mine, and I felt like I had a confidante again. We now live in different states, but our friendship and our kids' friendships have continued.

Connection is not just powerful, it is *essential* to us on every level, and we *have to* put the effort into finding it when we first get sober. This is why I suggest that many of my clients check out sober-support groups. Many people come into sobriety having burned a lot of bridges. Some of us still have friends, and some of us discover that what we actually have are fair-weather drinking buddies. Local sober-support groups can be a way to start rebuilding connection.

How has loneliness affected you?

Example: *I feel really lonely when I can't share what is really going on inside of me. I have often said yes to drinks even when I don't want to just for the company.*

How do you fuel your loneliness?

Example: *I know I have shut myself away from people and ignored their calls. Then they give up because I'm not giving them a response.*

Where could you start breaking down the walls of loneliness?

Example: *The groups I could join are _____. The people I could connect with are _____.*

...

SOBER-SUPPORT GROUPS

Many of you reading this book could benefit from sober-support groups. Particularly if you have recognized that your relationship with alcohol is abusive.

Getting sober is a massive lifestyle change. As you will see, boredom can be a factor in early sobriety. Most people tend to find they have a lot more time on their hands when drinking and recovering from drinking are no longer sucking up so much of their time. My weekends felt like gaping holes of time to fill—just hours and hours of not knowing what to do with myself. Going to a support group, hanging out afterward, and having coffee played a massive part in filling that time. Attending a support group also helped me understand that I really wasn't alone, that how I felt and my experiences with alcohol were actually very common. That's when sobriety felt possible to me.

Depending on where you live, it's likely that you have a variety of sober-support groups to choose from. I recommend that most of my clients try to find one when they first get sober. Apart from having a program, support, and socialization, meetings are places where we can go when we are struggling, where we don't have to pretend that everything is okay. We can drop the mask. Whatever sober-support group you go to, everyone who is there has felt the same way you do. You may not feel that when you walk in, but because they are there, you know they have been down the same road. We don't have to pretend that we are coping or that we are fine. A sober-support group is a place where it's possible to talk about what is really happening in your life and be listened to and understood. The key to exploring support meetings is to keep an open mind and keep showing up. We have to allow people to know us, and we can only do that if we attend regularly.

Sober support groups can offer so much to us when we stop drinking. They can make all the difference to our lives when we still feel raw and bruised from years of alcohol abuse. For a list of support groups, please check the "Resources" section at the back of the book. There you'll find a small taste of the different programs and services that have popped up or grown in membership since I got sober. Some are more prevalent online and have occasional in-person meetups, while some are just in person. However, since the COVID-19 pandemic, it's likely most of them now know how to offer both.

There are many more groups, particularly online. I would certainly caution you to do some due diligence before joining any group, particularly online ones. There are many people who have gotten sober and spotted business opportunities they wanted to exploit. Please make sure before purchasing any paid services that the people are qualified, experienced, and registered with the appropriate ethical body before committing your time and money. Many groups are generally peer led—often organized by volunteers and members—and they all differ in approach, philosophy, and access. This can be great, but it also can shield abusive and predatory behavior, which unfortunately can happen anywhere and in any kind of group. I want to say that most people in all groups are genuine and helpful. Find those people. Use good judgment, trust your gut instinct, and if someone feels predatory or unsafe, then practice boundaries. Find a senior group member and ask them for help and support.

In addition to sober-support groups, there are lots of wonderful sober social groups, like sober running clubs, sober book clubs, and sober meetups that you can find online. You could meet new people and know there would be no pressure to drink. I recently bought a Peloton, and there are several sober hashtags, so when I am in a class, I can see other sober people are there too. Sobriety has very much come out into the open. There is less stigma against and a growing movement for being alcohol-free as a lifestyle choice. I was reading an interview with teenage music phenomenon Billie Eilish the other day. She said she doesn't use alcohol or drugs (she's nineteen), not because she had a problem, but because she had seen lots of other people have problems, and it just didn't look attractive to her.[4] I love her attitude and that she is such a great role model for authenticity and how expansive a life can be without alcohol and drugs. Living alcohol-free is becoming a legitimate (and cool) lifestyle choice.

SOBRIETY: A FULL, FUN, PRODUCTIVE LIFE

The visibility of sober people from all walks of life is creating an atmosphere where being sober is becoming more normalized.

There are even sober bars popping up all over the place. I personally love the idea of sober bars (especially if there's dancing), because guess what—sober people also love to socialize and party! None of that needs to stop when you give up alcohol. Sober bars are providing ways to have fun where we don't have to deal with alcohol being in our faces or drunk people bothering us. More and more people are waking up to the fact that sobriety is fun.

One of the things I enjoy the most at large sober gatherings is watching people having fun sober. I especially enjoy the faces of the newly sober people the next morning as they walk around with a confused and perplexed expression on their faces. Their brains are still trying to wrap themselves around the idea that they had fun the night before—they danced, they chatted, they laughed and flirted. They went to bed with sore feet but not a sore head. They woke up in the right place without shame or embarrassment. It's baffling at first. *How was this possible without alcohol?* they wonder. They had a deeply ingrained belief that alcohol was required to have fun—you know, real fun. It was a fact, wasn't it? But here they are, having had real fun without alcohol. Who knew there was such a thing? And their beliefs about alcohol and what it brings begin to shatter. Their brain circuitry is rewiring itself as it expands into this new reality.

For me it's just funny, because I can remember what that felt like. I remember discovering, much to my relief, that I didn't have to give up anything but alcohol when I got sober. Quite the contrary—the dancing, the laughing, the socializing, and the fun were not just possible in sobriety, but were actually *better.* That just about blew my mind. After that there was no going back.

I want you to have this experience too. I want you to find your sober people and achieve a sense of belonging, and I want you to discover that you can have fun and you never need to be hungover again.

THE PATH TO CONNECTION IS THROUGH VULNERABILITY

To really understand connection, what it means, and how to achieve it, we can't avoid talking about vulnerability. Connection and vulnerability are intrinsically entwined. In fact, we can't achieve the connection we desire without it.

There is also a third component to this equation, and that is trust. Through vulnerability we create trust and connection. Vulnerability is an emotional risk we take to be truly seen. Being really seen (for who we are) is a basic human need.

Because I grew up in a family where I wasn't permitted to show any feelings or be vulnerable, I didn't feel seen. Because I didn't feel seen, I felt worthless and insignificant. I absorbed the idea that vulnerability and being seen were very bad things, so I created a hard shell around myself. I could not and would not show you what was really going on inside me. What I presented to the world was that I was okay, everything was okay, we are all okay. Let's not go any deeper than that. Who I was on the inside was different from who I presented on the outside. We call this incongruence. I was very concerned with what other people thought of me, and I presented what I thought they wanted to see. Vulnerability was a risk I just couldn't take. And this is how I lost my connection to myself—when I cut myself off from how I felt, I cut myself off from who I was.

Looking back, I can see now that even though I did manage to have some good friends around me when I was drinking, I never felt connected to them in the way I feel connected to my friends now because I didn't feel connected to myself. It was because I was unable to say how I was really feeling or show who I really was. If I couldn't do this with myself, how could I do it with anyone else? The idea of that was inconceivable and terrifying. I had too much pride and was terrified of being vulnerable. I thought it was a weakness. I didn't like who I was; I was uncomfortable in my own skin and I was deeply disconnected. When you can't be authentic, people can't really know you.

We don't just get these messages about vulnerability from our families, we get them from our culture too. It's embedded in cultural messages about what defines masculinity and femininity. Women may be permitted to show more vulnerability than men, but all of this is tightly restrained in cultural expectations of gender and race. Being vulnerable does not fit with the idea of masculinity, and men suffer hugely for it, pushing down all the feelings they are not "allowed" to have.

We believe alcohol makes expressions of vulnerability safer. But what we are creating is a façade of vulnerability rather than the real thing. Despite our fear of it, vulnerability calls us. There is something inside of us that is yearning for the real, to be seen as we are. And if we don't have the tools, then alcohol can feel like the answer to this. We can't risk exposing the realness inside of us without a filter or buffer. If we have had little practice at being vulnerable, then alcohol presents itself as a handy tool to make it more bearable. The struggle to be vulnerable is not just a problem for someone with an alcohol use disorder; it is a struggle of the human race.

This is why I am so grateful for Brené Brown's work on shame and vulnerability, and the global conversations she has ignited. This conversation hasn't arrived a moment too soon—we need to understand and tear down our limiting beliefs about vulnerability and start again. In *Dare to Lead*, she says, "What most of us fail to understand and what took me a decade of research to learn is that vulnerability is the cradle of the emotions and experiences we crave. Vulnerability is the birthplace of love, belonging, and joy."[5]

I mean that's just everything I've ever wanted. I thought alcohol was the best way to get it all, and it turns out it isn't; the best way was through vulnerability. Being vulnerable is a skill we can all learn, and something we must learn if we want to be sober.

Unlocking Vulnerability

One of the first steps in unlocking vulnerability is to challenge the stories we make up about ourselves and about being vulnerable. A lot of these would have come from our parenting. Think about the messages you were given from your parents about your feelings and emotions. If our parents didn't know how to handle their own emotions, they wouldn't have known how to handle ours. Typically, our feelings and emotions are suppressed or shut down in some way, and we learn not to bring this part of ourselves out in the open. This continues into adulthood and almost makes the abuse of alcohol (or other substances) *necessary*. If we can't fully express ourselves emotionally in the way we have been designed to, then we will suffer for it. And suffering is only tolerable for so long.

Vulnerability allows us to care for and nurture one another. There is nothing more sacred than being truly known in all our vulnerability. Vulnerability can bring out tenderness in other people because we all understand it. Watch how the temperature in a room changes when someone stops trying to "put on a facade" that everything is okay. We may have felt animosity toward that person or been indifferent to them, but when they are real and vulnerable there is *recognition*. And this recognition leads to connection. It leads to something real. When someone shows us what's inside of them, we realize that it's not that different from what's inside of ourselves, *no matter who they are*. We have this recognition because we are all the same inside. That's what's so crazy. We all feel and think very similar things. Everyone has limiting beliefs about themselves, and everyone feels shame and fear. Most people are afraid of vulnerability, so when we see people being vulnerable, it is reassuring, inspiring, and freeing because we are shown that vulnerability is *survivable*.

Vulnerability normalizes all of our experiences so we can see that we are not alone. I simply can't describe the relief you will feel when you know you are not alone in your suffering. It's not that the problem is necessarily solved right then, but the suffering becomes bearable when we know we are not the only person to feel or experience life in this way. It is the feeling of *aloneness* that is eating away at us. But when I see myself reflected in you, I feel just a little less alone and that is what leads to connection and healing. It is only through authentic connection that we can heal.

When people respond to our vulnerability, it confirms that our feelings and needs are valid and we are worth something. When we witness vulnerability in others, we need to respond with compassion and kindness. We need to place a value on other people's vulnerability and honor what we witness. Vulnerability can often be uncomfortable for others to witness. In fact, I've seen people try to shut down vulnerability in other people because they have found it to be uncomfortable. Vulnerability *will* feel uncomfortable. Accepting this instead of resisting it is easier in the long run. Because within the discomfort there is a lesson, and within the lesson there is growth, and we need all of these things to become free.

Taking Steps Toward Vulnerability

As you think about what vulnerability means to you, consider where and to whom you show it. Discernment is a skill: it's about trusting our inner guidance system to help us feel what is safe and what is not safe. What we need is an *empathetic witness* to what we are experiencing. An empathetic witness is not someone who judges us or even tries to fix us but someone who really hears and sees us and helps us reframe what we are going through.

The power of empathy is revolutionary. I remember trying to open up to a boyfriend (who I drank and used drugs with) about my panic attacks. I really needed help, and I tried to tell him how I felt. He laughed because of his own discomfort, and I felt like crap. He didn't help or support me and just compounded the feeling I had that I was weird. Of course, I ran his response through my filter system and connected it to the limiting belief that I wasn't good enough. None of those things were true. He was immature, and we were hungover. I chose a bad time and the wrong person, that's all. The next time I opened up about my panic attacks was with a sober woman who was loving and kind. I felt seen and supported. She didn't have any immediate solutions, but her support, kindness, and *empathy* were what I needed. I had found my first empathetic witness to my suffering. So, use your intuition and trust yourself when you begin to open up and reveal who you really are.

Lastly, shift your mindset as to what vulnerability means. We are given all these messages that vulnerability is a weakness when in fact it is a strength. There is truly only one path to meaningful connection and that is through vulnerability. This is the path you must take; there is no other way. It will scare you, but your life will be so much richer for it.

What beliefs do you have about vulnerability?

Example: *I've always believed it was a weakness and that you should try to cope with things on your own.*

Who do you have in your life that you could risk being vulnerable with?

Example: *I don't know, but I know I could talk to a therapist.*

...

CREATING THE CONNECTION WE NEED: THREE LEVELS OF CONNECTION

As we have discovered, there are three dimensions of loneliness. That means there are also three levels of connection. The depth of connection we have differs in each dimension. Psychologist Dr. Robin Dunbar described the need for three levels of friendship, with ourselves in the center. They are as follows: intimate/emotional, relational/social, and community.[6]

Level 1: Intimate/Emotional

The intimate/emotional level is typically connection with a smaller group of people, as it requires time and energy. It often occurs with an intimate partner, for example a romantic relationship, or a very close friend. The core of this connection is that the other person knows our soul. When someone knows our soul, we are truly seen and known, and this is a sacred and holy thing. It is a blessing to give and receive it. I think it is a mistake to believe that this can only happen with a romantic partner. This level of connection takes time, trust, and vulnerability, but it can exist in many forms.

When I met my husband, he introduced me to the Mountain Mamas. The Mountain Mamas were made up of his former stepmother and her two best friends. They had lived and worked together for over forty years. They are best friends and life partners but not romantic partners—their connection is deep, real, and platonic. At a certain point in all of their lives they each came to the decision that romance wasn't for them, but that they also wanted love, closeness, and connection. They are a sisterhood. They share everything equally and love and support each other. They are each other's family, and they are my extended family.

The Mountain Mamas live on a mountain near Los Gatos, California, and are completely self-sufficient. They have owned various businesses over the years and have lived and worked alongside each other in harmony. I have always loved and respected them and their journey, and how they have made a nontraditional arrangement and flourished within it. Each woman is held up and supported by the connection they have with the others. It is one of the greatest examples of meaningful connection I have ever seen.

Level 2: Relational/Social

The next level of connection we need is relational/social. This level is about having a circle of friends that we can grow with and relate to. As our circumstances change, our friends may also change. My husband joined a fraternity when he went to college. The young men he met there have been his closest friends for over four decades. Their college experience bonded them for life. They have regular meetups, and although sometimes geography and time make them challenging, I always want them to be a priority for my husband, as they just fill him up. I have four close friends from my drinking days who stuck by me, along with a lot of really good sober friends. I cherish what they bring to my life and work hard to carve out the time and space these relationships need in order to thrive and grow.

Once I became a mum, I began to have friends who had kids of a similar age. When I got sober, I was able to reconnect with my friends from college and high school. I was able to show up and be a good friend once alcohol wasn't getting in the way. You may also have friendships you have neglected, but once you have an honest conversation about what has been happening, you may find yourselves closer than ever. Friendships take time and energy and of course we have to balance all of this. But investing in friends is a dividend that will pay off over our lifetime.

Level 3: Community

We also need connection at the level of community—the feeling that we belong to a wider group. One of the wonderful things that the online sober community has given me is sober girlfriends. Our online connection has led to in-person friendships, and although none of us live nearby, we have visited one another and met up at some of the larger sober gatherings. Online connections are a good place to start and can turn into real-life connections. I am also involved in my kids' schools, the local drug prevention initiative, and local sober groups. All of this activity leads to a sense of belonging—a sense that we matter and we have something to contribute.

Journal Prompts to Create Connection

Are any of the three levels of connection missing for you?

Example: *Yes. I have a supportive partner, but I don't feel like I have many close friends or really feel part of my community.*

Have you had these missing levels in the past?

Example: *Yes. I used to coach my kid's soccer team and had lots of close friends through that and felt like I was doing something good in my community. But the hangovers on the weekend stopped all that.*

Have you explored any sober groups? What options are there for you locally?

Example: *AA scares me, but I have been to some online meetings, and I think I saw a sober running club nearby.*

...

THE JOURNEY OF CONNECTION

I hope in this chapter you have begun to understand what the real problem is and what is at stake. It's very easy to lose ourselves in an alcohol problem, but I want to emphasize that alcohol was never really the problem, it was just a symptom. It masked what was going on underneath and made it more bearable. Make connection your top priority. If your alcohol use has led to your being completely alone, then start with looking for a local sober-support group—they can be a safe harbor right now. Online support groups can also be very helpful and are sometimes an easier place to start. Or just reconnect with old friends or colleagues. Take a risk and reach out.

Also understand that there is probably a lot of negative self-talk going on in your mind right now. This voice is not the voice of truth; it's your critical voice. It is not real, but it will feel very powerful. This voice may try to talk you out of connecting. It may tell you all kinds of stories about why you can't connect with others. These stories aren't true. Use the five pillars to help you through this. Consciously creating connection is a key part of the sobriety process. Loneliness will eat away at us like a cancer and will take us back to a drink faster than anything else. Start small, start simply, but make sure you start. Show up consistently and allow people to know you. It takes time, but it will happen sooner than you think.

What is meaningful connection? It is when we have enough trust to be vulnerable, to show someone our broken parts, to have messy emotions and know they will still love and support us anyway. When we have meaningful connection with someone, it gives us grace in our process. Process work is rarely linear. It stops and starts and gets messy, and we make mistakes. As we grapple with emotions and understanding ourselves and the discomfort of change, meaningful connection can sustain us. As Vivek Murthy says, "It's in our relationships that we find the emotional sustenance and power we need in order to thrive. So strong is this instinct that when we move away from connection it induces genuine pain."[7]

Meaningful connection is food for our souls. Without it, we can't grow, and we can't be sober. The lack of connection is painful, and pain is one of the reasons we drink. So, we are presented with a choice: we can numb the pain or we can take the risk and make connection.

Choose connection.

Use these suggestions to uncover what connection means to you and how to increase connection in your life.

What have you learned about yourself from this chapter?
> Example: *It's really hit home how lonely I've been. I never saw it until now.*

What actions help you feel like you belong to yourself?
> Example: *Not drinking alcohol for sure. I want to like myself again by behaving in ways I'm not ashamed of.*

...

CHAPTER 7

The Pillar of Balance

When our relationship with alcohol no longer makes sense, we are out of balance. And frankly, it's not really possible to have balance in our lives when we use a carcinogenic substance[1] like alcohol on a regular basis. Our bodies have to continuously exert unnecessary energy to regain balance in our systems after we have been drinking even small amounts of alcohol. Because alcohol steals some of our bandwidth we don't operate with our full capabilities, so trying to balance your everyday needs while misusing alcohol is like swimming upstream. You will expend a lot of energy and not get very far. As our circumstances change, so do our needs, and balancing the two is a vital life skill, especially at the start of sobriety.

HALT—A USEFUL TOOL FOR BALANCE IN THE EARLY DAYS OF SOBRIETY

As we are discovering, balance is an art that changes and evolves over time, so balance a year from now will look different from what it is today. One of the best tools for learning balance in early sobriety is known as HALT,[2] a really handy acronym that stands for hungry, angry, lonely, and tired.

These are four powerful, common triggers that require our attention in a timely fashion before they take over and start calling the shots. When we abuse alcohol, we are not used to paying attention to our needs or to the messages our body is sending us. We are disconnected from ourselves, and our feelings become overwhelming; we resort to outside fixes like alcohol to quell those feelings. We also turn to food, screens, and consumerism. If we numb the negative feelings, we can ignore what being out of balance means for us. When we get sober, we have to learn new skills and tools—and one of these is listening and responding appropriately to the messages our bodies are sending.

Hungry

Our bodies need nutritious food on a regular basis. We all know this. It's not news, but we don't always make it a priority. Most of us can get pretty cranky if we are hungry. My husband and youngest son are prime examples of this. In the space of a few minutes, they can go from the gentle, loving creatures they normally are to full-on snappy rage monsters who need to be fed. You probably know someone like this too. And this stuff escalates fast. Disagreements, hurt feelings, and miscommunication occur—all things that have consequences we didn't intend.

As Abraham Maslow's hierarchy of needs explains, we can only take action based on which of our needs are being met. Physiological needs (food, water, warmth, shelter, sleep, and air) are the basis for meeting all our other needs (relationships, self-expression, belonging, and so on). We can't meet any of our other needs—or anyone else's either—if we are starving or thirsty. When we are like this, we can't learn or be patient or kind. Our physical hunger and thirst take over. Our bodies send us lots of hard-to-ignore signals that we need to meet these needs before anything else can happen.[3]

There are two things to learn here: start listening to your body when it is telling you to eat, and understand that the intense feelings that show up when you are hungry—like impatience, anger, and frustration—will usually disappear when you have eaten. It is often typical for my clients to have lost touch with their bodies and have really bad habits around food. Drinking too much does that. Our bodies crave salt and sugar when we are hungover. We don't have the time or the bandwidth to shop for and make healthy food, and we skip meals. Listening to our bodies and understanding not just that our bodies are hungry but what type of food they actually need and when, is the first step to getting balanced.

Tips for Managing the Hunger Trigger
- Carry snacks with you so if you do skip a meal you can at least refuel.
- Make small changes to what you eat; don't try drastic new diets.
- Practice listening to your body and the signals it is sending you. Are you thirsty? What are you hungry for?

Angry

The important thing to know about anger is that it is a normal and healthy emotion when appropriately expressed. It can fuel us, drive our actions, and be the root of change. We feel angry because of how we perceive certain situations, and how we experience that anger will be based on past experiences of those situations. Often, underneath our anger we feel wronged, threatened, powerless, or fearful. Anger flares up as a defense mechanism to deflect our attention from what is really going on, and it is usually quite scary for other people to experience, so it can be a handy weapon to keep people from getting too close.

Anger is often complicated, but it should never be ignored. If we don't use HALT to pay attention to the feeling of anger, we can express it in inappropriate ways that hurt ourselves and others. One of the worst ways we can deal with anger is to deny we are feeling it, push it down, and pretend it isn't there. This can then manifest in passive-aggressive behavior (saying one thing but meaning another), or it can turn inward as depression.

Anger can make drinking feel justified. When we have a complicated relationship with alcohol we are subconsciously looking for the "free drunk." By that I mean a reason to get drunk that you can blame on someone or something else. It's not *your* fault you got drunk; you *had* to have a drink because of what happened. It's the excuse we create to justify our actions to ourselves. Have you ever felt that way? I know I have. Righteous anger is in itself intoxicating, and my brain can do the necessary equations and convince me that what I do in response to that anger is not actually my fault. But in fact, what we are actually doing is creating a justification to have a drink or get drunk. Who pays the price? The person you are angry at? Nope.

We are allowed to be angry, but we want to pause and listen to the voice underneath, so we can understand what we are angry *about*, and what the appropriate next action is. Getting drunk or acting out our anger is not the next right action. Ever. When you wake up hungover the next day, has anything been achieved, resolved, or changed? Feel your anger and then go underneath it to find out what is being communicated. What is really happening? Get curious. This will feel hard at first but will be easier in the long run. We don't want to ignore our emotions; we want to gain mastery over them by understanding them. We can start by recognizing when we are angry, taking deep breaths, and then figuring out what's going on beneath the anger so we can choose a better response.

Tips for Managing the Anger Trigger
- Pay attention to your body and notice how the emotion shows up (a racing heart, feeling hot, and so on).
- Take deep breaths and say to yourself, *This is not an emergency. This is not personal.*
- Walk away if you can.
- When you feel calmer, journal about what happened so you can understand it better.

Lonely

This for me is the big one. Loneliness kills. We now have research that shows how loneliness affects not just our mental health but also our physical health.[4] One of the reasons we used to drink is that we believed alcohol promised us connection and belonging. This promise is a central message in nearly all of alcohol advertising. Who doesn't want to feel connection and belonging? We see images everywhere of people laughing, joking, and *connecting* while holding a drink in their hands. The link between alcohol and belonging is very powerful. I've had many clients who stumble because they are lonely, and they think alcohol is the answer to that because they believe it is required to socialize (it's not).

We are told and shown so many times that drinking alcohol will help us fit in, belong, and feel connected to others. But when our experience does not always match the messaging, we don't conclude that the messaging is wrong. Instead we think it's our fault and that if we could just manage our drinking better, we would capture the feelings alcohol promises. Sometimes we achieve this feeling of connection and belonging through alcohol, but we discover that it actually has a steep price. Alcohol, and more importantly the repercussions of drinking alcohol, make us feel not just farther apart from others but disconnected from ourselves and lonelier than ever.

Take this one seriously. It is not as easily solvable as hunger, but it absolutely cannot be ignored. Loneliness can often feel shameful, as if we are defective or there is something wrong with us. This feeling of shame will make us want to withdraw and not be seen, thus compounding the feeling of loneliness. In this way loneliness becomes a cancer that keeps spreading.

The first step is to recognize how lonely we are. I feel it is an act of bravery to acknowledge one's loneliness. It feels like a punch to the gut when we realize we have somehow maneuvered ourselves to a place where we are closed off from people.

Once you have recognized that you are lonely, start creating a plan to connect with people. Sobriety groups can be particularly helpful when you are at this stage, as you don't have to pretend that everything is okay. No one walks into a recovery meeting because everything is going well. I believe we can find compassion and companionship in sober-support meetings—even if only for a little while—and that can go a very long way in helping us feel less alone.

Religious organizations and community groups can also provide you with company, as can meditation, exercise, and book clubs where there isn't such an emphasis on drinking. Volunteering for a cause that feels purposeful is also a great way to meet new people. If we look around we will find that there are many things we could do to connect with others. When we feel lonely, we don't feel *seen* by others, and we feel like we don't matter. We do matter, and we must summon our courage to go somewhere where we can receive a kind word or hello. Being seen in this way is incredibly powerful, but the responsibility is on you to take the steps.

Tips for Managing the Lonely Trigger
- Tell yourself that loneliness isn't a moral failing on your part.
- List all the people you like who you could reach out to.
- Reach out in the way that feels most comfortable for you (text, email, phone call).
- Make a commitment to meet a friend or go to a group of some kind.

Tired

Learning balance is all about learning to manage our energy. We don't function well when our resources are depleted. We can feel tearful, vulnerable, and overwhelmed. Everything just feels like too much, and every task is much, much harder than it needs to be. We cannot show up for our families, our work, or ourselves if we are exhausted.

I know life is busy, but this is not a state we can tolerate for very long. We have to rest, have downtime, and get enough sleep, otherwise we burn ourselves out and feel uncomfortable, and our brains start thinking of alcohol as a solution.

In her book *The Sleep Revolution: Transforming Your Life, One Night at a Time*,[5] Arianna Huffington points out how our attitude toward sleep undermines our lives and what we produce. Sleep is not valued in our culture, and there is a competitiveness around sleeping less and working more. Huffington zeroes in on how this attitude is literally undoing us. I believe that the need to rest or sleep is seen as a weakness, which is why we don't prioritize it. Getting enough sleep and proper rest, however, is how we succeed and do more, and it is another skill we need to learn. Although I have always been strict about my sons' bedtime, they will still use delaying tactics to postpone it. I'm wise to all of them, and they don't work with me, but then I see myself doing the same thing when it's time for me to go to bed. I'll just check my phone or watch the news quickly or start a task that could really wait until morning. It's called bedtime procrastination, and while there are many reasons we do it, it always results in our not getting enough rest.

Of course, many people use alcohol to help them sleep. Alcohol doesn't help us sleep better (you knew that, right?); it interferes with our circadian rhythm and affects the quality of our sleep. In fact, alcohol may have been keeping us from getting a good night's rest for years. It will take a while for our bodies to adjust, and we may even experience insomnia or fatigue when we first get sober.

There is much we can do to manage how tired we are. It's not just about getting enough sleep; it's managing where and how we spend our energy, so we don't burn ourselves out. It's balancing the things we have to accomplish in one day and the tasks we say no to. It's giving ourselves permission just to chill out and relax—to leave tasks half done because our energy levels are low. This is balance, and it will look different day to day and week to week.

Tips for Managing the Tired Trigger
- Research and practice sleep "hygiene" (don't have screens in the bedroom, reduce or eliminate caffeine, and so on).
- Observe where your energy gets drained. What could you change?

HALT SUMMARY

When we feel hungry, angry, lonely, or tired we will also feel uncomfortable. HALT is really about data that we need to pay attention to. It serves as a warning signal, and all humans get them—it's just that we're not great at responding to and processing them. We can all tolerate some discomfort, but because we have successfully trained our brains to look for quick external fixes to internal problems, feeling any element of HALT is particularly dangerous to people in early sobriety.

Learning how to respond to the elements of HALT is our first step into learning emotional sobriety and staying in balance.

Further Steps to Responding to Hunger, Anger, Loneliness, and Tiredness

- Stop. Notice the sensations in the body.
- Breathe. Pay attention to the feelings.
- Take a guess as to what is going on. Ask yourself questions like, *What is this feeling? Where am I out of balance? What do I need right now?*
- Go over the HALT triggers and see if one fits. Accept what is happening.
- Ask yourself what the next right action would be to change this. Take the next right action.

We are purposefully choosing a different response, one that benefits us rather than harms us. Like all things, it will take practice. Using alcohol as a response to feeling hungry, angry, lonely, or tired is a conditioned response, but we can learn other conditioned responses. This is the work of early sobriety.

In addition to HALT I want to add three more triggers that you should be aware of: stress, boredom, and hormones.

Stress

When the body experiences or perceives stress, it provokes a biological response. We can experience stress in our stomachs, our central nervous systems, and our brains. We also know that long-term exposure to stress can be a contributing factor to disease and sickness.[6] However, none of us can avoid stress; it is a part of life.

Our response to stress is programmed into us. If we are in a dangerous situation, the fight-or-flight response is triggered in our brains. We need this response to help us act quickly to avoid danger. Even if the danger is not an actual threat but only perceived as one, the stress response is still triggered. Prolonged stress is uncomfortable and disturbing, as our bodies were not designed to handle it.

In our modern lives we can all experience many external stress triggers. We may not have the power to eliminate all of these triggers, but in cases where we do have control, we should take steps to reduce or remove the stressor. In many cases it's really more about how we choose to respond to stress, recognizing how much is self-inflicted and making changes where we can.

While it is clear that we can't avoid stress, we do need to find better ways to manage it. Balance in our lives is key here. We need to balance our priorities, our needs, other people's needs, and our energy levels. If we overcommit ourselves, then not only do we end up exhausted, we also feel stressed, and these are two risk factors for drinking. Many of us have used alcohol to deal with stress; in fact, I would say it is encouraged as an acceptable method of doing so. Unfortunately, alcohol doesn't help with stress at all. In fact, it makes things worse. In early sobriety, we need to look at where we are adding unnecessary stress to our lives. What can you reduce right now? Are you taking on too much? Are you afraid to say no?

Stress, like anger, is not necessarily a bad thing. It is designed to keep us alive by keeping us alert to danger. But we can no longer use alcohol to manage it.

Tips to Manage the Stress Trigger

- Ask yourself, *Does this need to be done now? Does it need to be done by me? Will the world end if I don't get it done?* Often our stress is due to our inner monologue and pressure we put on ourselves. Sometimes things don't need to be done right now or even by us, and they often don't have to be done perfectly, if at all.
- If you are in a stressful job, look for where you can ask for help, delegate, or manage your energy better. Have you taken on too much?
- Be aware of how you spend and give your time. Are you giving too much and running on empty? Are you spending too much time with people who drain your energy?

Boredom

I wanted to add boredom to the list of triggers in early sobriety as I hear about it a lot in my Facebook group and from newly sober folks. It is one of the initial obstacles we have to navigate past. Never has this been more apparent than during the COVID-19 pandemic, when so many of our avenues for entertainment and community have been closed. Alcohol use and abuse has risen dramatically, and a big reason is boredom. Our days have lacked structure and connection, and we have filled these gaps with alcohol. Did you drink during lockdown because it felt like there was nothing else to do?[7]

Some days sobriety will feel tedious. I remember being a few months sober and cleaning my apartment from top to bottom on a Saturday night because I literally didn't know what else to do. And I remember thinking, *Is this it?* I'm only twenty-seven years old. Is my life always going to be this boring? But I want to say that the problem isn't boredom, its perspective. Alcohol can take up a lot of time and energy, and when we quit, we have time to fill. We have to learn how to get to The Land—the one of fun, excitement, belonging, connection, relaxation, rewards, and romance—without using alcohol. I kid you not: I literally had no idea how to manufacture fun without the aid of booze.

When I stopped drinking, the weekend and evenings felt like they stretched on forever. I had to learn how to build a new life. After the first year of sobriety (when I was twenty-eight) I was doing all the things any twenty-eight-year-old was doing. I was socializing, going to clubs and concerts, dancing, going on dates, taking vacations, and having barbeques. I did all of them sober, and all of them were better because of it. As I got older I did different things for fun, and not one of them would have been a better experience by adding alcohol to it. But you have to give yourself the space for this to happen, as it takes a little time. Getting sober is a lifestyle shift. It will feel odd at first. Alcohol can make our lives feel smaller, because it's just repeating the same experience over in a different bar. The world is so rich; there is so much to do and discover if we only look.

It wasn't always like this. Long ago you did different things that didn't require alcohol for their enjoyment. Find those things, and start doing them again. Find new things to try to fill time as best you can with as many supportive activities as possible. Keep putting your energy into the stuff that is fulfilling and joyful. Accept that this is a process and there is no quick fix, but know that you are part of a global community of people who are all at different stages of doing this. Work on it, and I promise it will change. I can't remember the last time I felt bored or had time to fill; my life is full and diverse. You will get there too, but you have to purposefully build it.

Tips to Manage the Boredom Trigger

- Identify the times when you feel bored. Is it in the evening or on weekends? Plan ahead. Schedule activities or connections at those times.
- Seek out new activities. If it's available, try going to a yoga or meditation class on a Friday night.
- Make sure you have plans for the weekend, even if it's just a support meeting or a walk with a friend. Small activities will grow into bigger, more fulfilling ones.

Hormones

Hormonal changes can have an impact on our quest to stop drinking. I have seen many women struggle to do everything right but who are defeated by hormonal fluctuations, especially in the early days. Women are more susceptible to mood disorders such as depression, anxiety, and sleeplessness due to fluctuating estrogen levels.[8] If you have PMS or are perimenopausal or menopausal and are *also* five days sober then you are going to experience additional challenges. You will have to deal with all the triggers of early sobriety plus raging hormones and that means you may need an extra layer of support. I would strongly suggest that all women seek help from their health-care provider and a nutritionist to understand what is happening in their bodies at different times of the month and as they age. With this knowledge and insight, women can increase their chances of successfully staying sober.

Tips to Manage the Hormones Trigger

- It's really important for women to learn about their own bodies. Get a full health checkup with blood work.
- Research or work with a professional who can help you make changes to manage hormone fluctuations better.

- Keep track of your cycle so you know when fluctuations will occur.

Journal Prompts to Create Balance in Early Sobriety

What is the biggest trigger for you? Hunger, anger, loneliness, tiredness, stress, boredom, hormones?

> Example: *Definitely anger, but I also get depressed before my period is due.*

What happens when you don't take care of these needs?

> Example: *When I feel angry, I just blow up at whomever is around me. And PMS is always a trigger.*

What small change could you make to feel more balanced?

> Example: *I need to listen more and not take things so personally. I'm going to speak to my doctor about how I can support myself better.*

...

CREATING BOUNDARIES, CREATING BALANCE

Boundaries and balance are very closely related. In order to have balance in our lives, we have to practice boundaries. Having a boundary is what gives us space and room to create balance in our lives—to identify our needs and respond to them. Having boundaries is not selfish. Rather, it enables us to balance our own needs so that we can manage our energy and show up for the people we care about and the things that matter in our lives. Unfortunately, creating boundaries is a life skill that most of us missed out on learning. Ideally, it should be role modeled in our homes, but a lot of us didn't grow up seeing healthy boundaries being set, so we picked the skill up by trial and error. As a result we have inadequate boundaries, no boundaries, or boundaries that we implement in a hurtful way. In *Rising Strong*, Brené Brown says, "Setting boundaries means getting clear on what behaviors are okay and what's not okay."[9] I never knew such a concept even existed until I got sober. I had no idea what a boundary was, that I was allowed to have them, or how to implement them. The idea of setting a boundary with other people simply blew my mind.

A lot of our problems, and I mean a *lot*—including setting in motion chains of events we don't like and forcing us to have difficult and uncomfortable interactions with people—come from our inability to set boundaries. Trust me when I say that learning to have boundaries will change your life.

Entrenched Beliefs

Before we get into how to set boundaries, I want to explain why it can feel so difficult at first (and it will). Many of us were raised to believe that we are responsible for how other people feel or that our own feelings are insignificant. When we have these beliefs, we can't have boundaries. We can have one or the other but not both. Letting go of these beliefs isn't going to happen overnight. It is a process of unlearning deeply entrenched behavior. Most of these behaviors are automatic and tied to beliefs hidden in our subconscious mind that we have no idea about.

When we think we're responsible for other people's feelings, we believe we have to modify, adapt, and change our behavior so that others are happy, or so they'll find us acceptable. What makes this challenging is that we really have no idea what other people's feelings truly are, so we are guessing. This takes up an enormous amount of energy and bandwidth. We can tie ourselves up in knots. And here's the kicker: despite all that energy and effort, we still may not make the other person happy. Then we feel like we have failed.

The first step in changing this situation is accepting that it isn't your job to make other people happy. I know for some people that can feel like a revolutionary and earth-shattering statement. When we have built our identity around pleasing others and discover that this has been a mistake, the ground shifts beneath our feet.

It does not mean that we don't *care* about how other people feel or that their feelings don't matter. It's that we are responsible for *our* emotional experience, and *others* are responsible for *theirs*. I take responsibility for my feelings by choosing my responses and by maintaining healthy boundaries.

The other faulty belief is that our own feelings don't matter. This belief can come from our childhood conditioning. Maybe we were told to quit crying about something that made us upset, or to "just get over it." Maybe our feelings were ignored, minimized, or brushed away. The lesson we would learn from this as a child would be *don't have feelings, your feelings don't matter*. My family didn't "do" feelings; feelings made everyone uncomfortable. It was explicitly and implicitly communicated to us that it was unacceptable to discuss our feelings and that we should shut them down. So I stuffed all of mine inside, and they sat like a powder keg within me. I didn't know how to listen to them or respond to them. My feelings were a foreign country, and I didn't speak the language. I was emotionally illiterate and therefore incapable of having boundaries. I was also conditioned to believe that I had to make my mother happy and only do things she would approve of. This then carried over into my adult relationships, and I would agonize over things I said or did and whether I was approved of or liked.

Learning to have boundaries with others is not just a foundation stone to sobriety, it's essential for life as a human being. Do not skip this step.

How to Set Boundaries

My favorite way to teach boundaries is by using the rule "Say what you mean, mean what you say, but don't say it mean." I believe this came from the Alcoholics Anonymous fellowships, but I'm not certain. Using this rule changed my life. It really is perfect in every way. When you are first practicing boundaries, it really helps to have a firm structure to hold on to. Communication with others can be a messy business when feelings are involved (as they usually are), and there are so many ways we can miscommunicate, causing harm and triggering a whole set of unnecessary problems. This rule will help you and keep others safe.

Let's break it down.

Say What You Mean

We can practice being precise with our words. Other people do not need long-winded explanations, they need clarity. If someone asks you to help out with something, and you can't or don't want to for whatever reason, don't launch into a rambling story about all the things you have to do, or that you want to help but you're not sure if you are free, and so on. The reason we do this is that we are scared to say no, and we are trying to soften it by overexplaining. Instead of saying, "I'm not sure, maybe. I have to get home for the dog, and I don't know what time my partner will be home, but if they are home early I could," say, "I'm sorry, I'd love to help, but I'm not free then," or "I have to check and get back to you." Get to the point; don't waste words and don't tell unnecessary stories. When we launch into a lengthy explanation we weaken the boundary we are trying to set by not being clear.

Mean What You Say

Our yes needs to mean yes, and our no needs to mean no. Do not agree to do things that you have no intention of doing or that you are going to back out of.

The reason people say yes when they actually mean no is because of the faulty belief that they are responsible for the other person's feelings. They believe that if they say no, the other person will be hurt, disappointed, upset, or angry, and that will be their fault. Because we think we're responsible for those feelings, we say things we don't mean. This makes us a liar and a thief (I'll explain that bit in a second).

Personally, I love a no. I'm more than happy with a no. Then I know exactly where I stand, and I can move on to plan B. What I can't stand is a wishy-washy yes—a yes that I suspect isn't firm and won't be followed through on. Then I am spending energy worrying whether you are going to do the thing you said you would do, or whether you are going to let me down at the last minute. Now, I may be disappointed, hurt, or upset with your no, but those are my feelings that I have to take responsibility for. I just want to know where I stand so that I can respond accordingly.

There is also another level to this. When we believe we have to be responsible for other people's feelings, it leaves us open to manipulation. Other people can sense that we can be manipulated and will exploit our need to please and not to hurt feelings. You may recall times when you have felt manipulated into doing something you didn't want to do. It probably left you feeling angry, hurt, or used. The reason that this happens is that we leave ourselves open to manipulation—in many cases, we have actually volunteered for it. This is why boundaries are so important. They protect us and keep this kind of thing from happening.

All human beings are trying to get their needs met. We will do this by whatever method works. If manipulating others gets me what I want, then I will keep doing it because it works. When it stops working, I will be forced to try something different.

The other thing to keep in mind is that *we teach other people how to treat us.* If people can tell (and they can) that we can be "guilted" into doing something, then they will use that tactic. It's not because they are bad people; it's because it works. Manipulating people is laziness. It's not a relationship-building tactic, it's a "getting what I want" tactic. Manipulative people will seek out those they know can be manipulated. The wonderful thing is that once you have boundaries, they don't come anywhere near you because they sense that it's not worth the effort.

Don't Say It Mean

The scariest part about creating boundaries, if we are not used to it, is that it can make us feel like a bad person. Not everyone will be happy about our boundaries, and they may show feelings of hurt and disappointment or have other negative reactions. We may feel very shaky when we first witness this happening (this shaky feeling is known as afterburn, and we will discuss how to deal with this a bit later), but the potential for a negative reaction is precisely why this rule is so brilliant and keeps everybody safe. *How* you say things really matters. It's important that we communicate with compassion and integrity. We want to be calm and clear; we don't want to insult or cause injury. The "how you say it" part is where we *can* have responsibility for hurting someone's feelings. If I state my boundary in a rude, aggressive, spiteful, or mean way, then I have played a part in causing someone pain. However, if I am clear about what I am communicating and say it precisely and in a calm and compassionate manner, then I am not responsible for how the other person receives that information, and I have taken responsibility for the emotional experience I want to have in the interaction.

***

There are a couple of extra elements that we need to bear in mind when we begin practicing how to have boundaries: repetition and afterburn.

Repetition

When you first start practicing boundaries, you need to expect to repeat them several times. There are several reasons for this.

The first one is that you have taught other people what to expect from you. *You* may know you have changed, but it is going to take other people a while to catch up. At first, they won't even really hear what you said, as they won't be expecting it. When you use the rule, keep it very simple and expect to repeat what you have said (with only minor variations) several times.

I had this experience at the beginning with a couple of family members. They tried numerous different ways to get me to do what it was they wanted, but I stuck to the rule and just kept repeating it. I didn't get angry or frustrated, because I knew this was a process and it would take time for everyone to adjust. The key here is to stay calm and know that how the other person is reacting isn't personal. They have been used to things being one way for a long time, so they will be confused at first. Stick to the rule of "don't say it mean." We don't want to undo the boundary we are trying to set.

When we repeat our boundaries, it's also important to keep saying the same thing as simply as possible. A mistake we can make is that when someone pushes back on our boundary, we then launch into a story as to why we can't do the thing they want. When we do this, we open doors that the other person will exploit. "Oh, you can't do Friday, okay I get it, but you could do Saturday? Let's do that!" And then before you know it you have found yourself agreeing to the thing you didn't want to do anyway. Explanations and stories leave you wide open for that. The other thing to remember is that people do not need to hear your story of "why." Yes, in some cases, with certain relationships, this would be appropriate if it helps someone understand. But in a lot of cases, this is really unnecessary. Telling the story is a trap, so be prepared to repeat your boundary several times, stay calm, and know that it is just taking the other person a while to realize things have changed. Stick to the rule every time.

Afterburn

It is very typical that after using the rule to set a boundary, we experience afterburn. Afterburn is the feeling you experience when your boundary has been heard and the other person walks away disappointed or upset that you can't do the thing that they want you to do. All kinds of thoughts crash in: *I'm a terrible person. Do they hate me now? What will other people think? Did I do the right thing? Will they still like me?*

Taking responsibility for our own emotional experience is a new and strange feeling. We may have set a boundary that causes someone to feel hurt and upset. If you used the rule and didn't "say it mean," then you haven't caused them hurt, but it will still feel like you did.

Rescuing other people from their uncomfortable feelings can be a hard habit to break. All we need to do is say, "Sure, no problem, I can do it," and the other person's face lights up and they are happy. But, and this is a big but, we have then made ourselves miserable. I can say yes and then spend days regretting and feeling miserable and resentful because I have agreed to something I didn't want to do. This is what I mean when I say we are responsible for our own emotional experience. If I do not want the emotional experience of feeling upset and resentful—and wasting time trying to think of how I can get out of something—then I need to be responsible for setting a boundary.

When our yes means yes and our no means no, we create space and calm in our lives. I can show up and help people, be of service, and meet my commitments because I am managing my energy and emotions. Having boundaries is not about never being helpful or of service to others; it's about making sure I can show up when I say I will and having the energy to do the things I committed to. When I say yes to everything for fear of upsetting someone, I will burn myself out, do a bad job, or just let that person down at the last minute because in reality I just don't have the energy to do all those things they are asking of me.

The afterburn will hit in the beginning. It will feel uncomfortable, but there are lots of tools, like journaling or talking it through with someone, to help us process that. The afterburn will go away; it won't stay around forever. In fact, you will find that it decreases over time and is a much easier experience than the feeling of agreeing to something you didn't want to do, then spending days agonizing about how to get out of it, as feelings of frustration and resentment grow. This is how we take responsibility for our emotional experience.

Thieves and Liars

When we don't have good boundaries, we become thieves and liars. This may feel a little uncomfortable—who wants to think of themselves this way? But clearly, when we say yes but really mean no, we are lying. We are misleading people and that is dishonest. But did you know that when we behave this way, we also become thieves too? When we allow ourselves to be manipulated by people because we are scared of causing hurt feelings, what we are also doing is stealing a growth opportunity from them.

Here's why. As I said, manipulation is lazy, but people use it because it works. If someone hasn't ever needed to develop different skills to get their needs met, then why would they? However, if manipulation stops working, maybe that person would be forced to think, *Huh, what am I going to do now?* And that is a chance for them to grow. What we steal when we are not honest is a growth opportunity for someone else. Don't take that away from them.

Journal Prompts to Start Having Better Boundaries

Who do you need to have boundaries with?

Example: *My mother and sister!*

What happens in this relationship when you don't have boundaries?

Example: *I feel angry and resentful. They never listen to me or consider what I want. It's always about them and what they want to do, and I just have to go along with it.*

How do you want this relationship to be different?
> Example: *I want to say no to some of the things they ask me to do, so I can say yes to the things I enjoy with them. I want to enjoy my time with them without feeling like I am going to explode.*

...

THE BALANCE PLATE

Imagine a plate divided up into sections with each section representing one of the following human needs:

- Purpose (career/work)
- Emotional and mental health
- Spiritual health
- Physical health
- Family, friends, and social life
- Passions, hobbies, and interests

We all have variations of these needs. They will differ from person to person and are based on our particular circumstances and our privileges. Our job is to learn how to balance these needs, just like balancing food on our plate. When our food gets out of balance, we know about it pretty quickly.

WHATEVER THE QUESTION, BALANCE IS ALWAYS THE ANSWER

Balance is an art, and while we will never be perfect at it, it is the practice of it that matters.

Our needs change as our circumstances change. Often, we don't always notice this and are uncomfortable for longer than necessary. Feeling discomfort, or feeling uncomfortable in our own skin, is usually a warning that something is out of balance, and we need to pay attention. Pausing and reflecting on what needs are not getting met is the first step to feeling better and protecting our sobriety.

We can't stay out of balance for very long. It just feels too uncomfortable and then triggers a whole set of other problems that compound the original issue. The first thing to check is the HALT triggers. Then we can move on to the deeper work.

I want to break these needs down so we can look at them more closely. But before I do, I want to talk about privilege. The ability to balance our needs is still dependent on how privileged we are. I'm aware that there is inequality in what we can access in order to meet our needs. While some have easy access to health care, education, and job opportunities, others do not. Balance is about taking responsibility for what you can change. For those of us who have more opportunity, privilege, and access, our job is to fight for this imbalance to be righted for everyone else.

Let's have a look at some of the things that affect our balance.

Purpose (Career/Work)

It's about what gets us up in the morning—to pay the rent, sure, but also to give our lives meaning. I know this is one of the areas that often feels most out of balance for people. Most of us have experienced working in a job that kills our souls. It becomes completely consuming and can take over our whole lives. I think for many people, feeling happy and fulfilled in their employment is a luxury born of privilege. I also think that everything can get better in sobriety no matter what your current circumstances. It doesn't mean it's going to change overnight. We all have to pay our bills, and change in this area can often feel very slow. However, when we start practicing the pillar of movement and understand what our values are, then we can begin to match those values to what we do or move toward what it is we wish we could do in the world.

Emotional and Mental Health

Taking care of our emotions and mental health is crucial to sobriety. How we feel is the driving force of what we do, so taking care of our emotions is paramount. It's very common for my clients to experience depression and anxiety, as well as other complex mental health issues. Alcohol causes and exacerbates mental health conditions. For some people, anxiety and depression will begin to disappear once they get sober and begin to take care of themselves. Others will need support from mental health professionals.

There is a very close relationship between addiction and mental health challenges. It's often hard to see which came first, as substance abuse can often be a form of self-medicating an underlying mental health challenge. Learning to take care of our emotional needs is a lifetime practice. We often go from being completely cut off from our emotions to having them flood us when we get sober. It can feel overwhelming. Getting expert support wherever possible is my best advice. There are so many types of therapy to help deal with anxiety, panic attacks, depression, and more.

Some people are blessed with a seemingly balanced disposition. But if you are anything like me, you have to work at it. I have much more awareness now of the things that can impact my mental and emotional health, and I'm much better at taking action earlier, so that I can mitigate their impact. Sobriety allows us to build self-awareness so we can learn these lessons. Learn to listen to your body and the messages it is sending you; pay attention and respond as best you can. I often find that a simple response, like speaking to someone, journaling, or going to a support meeting, can make the world of difference to how I feel.

Spiritual Health

If you have listened to my podcast you know that my cohost Chip Somers is a card-carrying atheist. Yet he is one of the most spiritual people I know.

It takes time, curiosity, and self-compassion to understand what spirituality means to us, and how we meet our spiritual needs is very personal. If you think of your spirit as the essence of who you are inside, our spirit is our soul, and spirituality is just being good to our souls as much as we can. It is paying attention to what we feed our souls. I understand spirituality as the "knowing" inside of me. This inner guidance system is where my values come from. When I got sober, I realized that honoring that spirit inside of me was the most important job I had. It is yours too.

Physical Health

We can only ignore our health and physical well-being for so long. Every human being needs the basics of sleep, exercise, food, and water. Not getting enough sleep for days or weeks on end will affect our immune system, cognitive function, and mood. We also need to eat right, exercise, and get treatment for any ongoing health problems. Pain management is an important part of this, and I have had many clients use alcohol to manage pain or discomfort in their bodies. Seeking out the right treatment and support is crucial to be successful in sobriety. Alcohol can really interfere with our body's natural functions, so when we don't drink we have a better chance of tuning in to what our bodies need.

Family, Friends, and Social Life

This is really about our need for connection—for meaningful human connection with people we care about and who fill us up. How we get these needs met is wildly different. My best friend is an introvert. She is very sociable and fun, but after a certain amount of time with other people she needs to then spend several days on her own, replenishing her energy.

The basic difference between introverts and extroverts is where they get their energy from.[10] Introverts get energized from spending time in solitude. Extroverts get energized from being with people. I'm an extrovert. I am also an only child, so I can manage solitude quite well, but I do love being around people too. Now, of course we can be around people a lot and still feel disconnected and lonely if we feel our connection needs are not being met. As we have seen, when loneliness shows up, it is a clear signal that we need to connect with someone in order to meet these needs. However, we also need to have boundaries.

Having a family limits how much time we can spend with our friends. But to stay balanced and healthy within our family, we also need to spend time with our friends and have time when we can be ourselves and not just someone's parent or partner. We can feel pulled in a lot of different directions and balancing that takes work and boundaries.

Sometimes we have to stop and look at who is making demands on our time. I have a client who cares for elderly parents, which she is happy to do, but it also depletes her energy. Balancing her needs and having boundaries has meant she is less resentful and tired, and she is more available to help her parents.

Passions, Hobbies, and Interests

I think this need can be described simply as "what lights us up." It might be gardening, going to church, dancing, reading more books, walking on the beach, spending time with people we like, or helping others. It's the thing that fills us with purpose and gives our lives meaning. It's about fun and finding pleasure in life. Don't think this is an insignificant need; it's not. In many ways it's a self-care need; it's a little something for yourself. If you dislike your job, then this need is doubly important as it's what brings meaning to your life. I learned to ski at age forty-seven. It was terrifying, but I wanted to do it as my kids were learning, and I wanted us to ski as a family. We get up early on the weekends and hit the slopes by 8:30 a.m.—something that never would have been possible with a hangover! The great thing about not drinking is that it opens up all sorts of opportunities to do and try things you never would have done or tried while you were drinking. We can create space in our lives by not drinking, and it can be filled with all sorts of incredible things.

A LIFETIME PRACTICE

Balance is something we will practice for the rest of our lives. As our circumstances change so do our needs. Getting sober is a big change in our circumstances, and what it means to us in the first year is different from what it will mean in our second, and so on. The point being that our circumstances will continue to change and so will our needs. With practice we will get better at reading the signals that tell us we are out of balance. Our bodies will give us clues that we will become more tuned in to. When we notice these signals we need to ask ourselves, *Where am I out of balance?* Often we already know the answer; we have just been ignoring it. Once it comes to our attention, we need to take action to restore balance.

Journal Prompts to Manage
Our Balance Plate

Which need on the balance plate feels most out of balance for you right now?

> Example: *Right now it feels like family. I'm not connecting with my kids; I'm just marshaling them through the day. I'm missing things and I don't want that. I want to cherish my time with them.*

What changes do you need to make to feel more balanced?

> Example: *I am doing too much and am so stressed. Half the stuff I worry about doesn't matter. I am going to learn to say no to things, so I can say yes to the stuff that energizes me.*

How does lack of balance show up in your body?

> Example: *I get insomnia and can't sleep.*

What tools can you use to manage balance better?

> Example: *I am going to practice listening to my body, instead of ignoring the sensations. I am going to try to recognize what my body is telling me.*

...

CHAPTER 8

The Pillar of Process

I want you to know that you matter. Everything you have gone through, everything you have felt, all that has made you who you are—I want you to know all of that matters. Now, I can tell you this, and you can say, "Yeah, that's great, thanks." But what I'm going to guess you'll do next is dismiss it or think it's irrelevant or, worse, that it doesn't actually apply to you.

Here is why I don't want you to do that. To really move on, we have to matter to *ourselves*. Otherwise we are just getting in our own way. Process work is about validating, honoring, feeling, processing, and accepting what happened in the past, so you can move on. Because what happened to you matters. Our past shapes our present. None of us can escape that.

The reason we have to do process work is that it's hard to make sense of things when we are in the middle of them. We absorb the feelings and messages without fully understanding them. Process work can only be done on reflection and in hindsight. But instead of reflecting on our process—Why did I feel that way? Why did I act that way? What do I think that means about me?—we distract or numb.

Process work is about understanding our feelings and emotions and to do that we have to be open and vulnerable, which is why we resist. If all we are doing is distracting and numbing, then we are not growing emotionally the way we are capable of. We will be emotionally stuck, getting older but not wiser. The work of really knowing ourselves and healing our past is universal. Everyone has to do it. However, the motivation to do this work really only comes from pain. I think distraction, busyness, and substance abuse are all methods people use to avoid self-reflection. Which is why I want you to see this as a gift. If you are changing your relationship with alcohol, then this is an invitation to process and let go of behaviors and feelings that no longer serve you. People talk about "freedom" a lot in relation to sobriety, and I want to be clear about what that really means. Of course, it applies to never feeling like you need or want a drink, but the greater implication is the freedom to access all our bandwidth. *It's freedom in our minds.*

Our thinking can get tangled, and we can burn a lot of energy going around in circles repeating the same mistakes from the past. When we understand ourselves better, we stop sabotaging our growth. That is freedom. The pillars of process and growth are entwined. We have to grow emotionally (that never stops), and we can only do that through really understanding what makes us tick. One of the most common ways that we demonstrate patterns from our past is in our relationships with other people. We subconsciously repeat patterns, because we don't understand why we feel the way we do when we are in relationships. Every relationship we have is really an invitation to grow.

THE PAST SHOWS UP IN OUR PRESENT

I understand why this is uncomfortable to think about. I have often heard the following from clients: "I don't want to go raking up the past" or "The past is the past—it doesn't matter now" or "I don't want to talk about stuff that happened a long time ago."

What my clients are actually saying is that they are scared. Whether it was ten or fifty years ago, the pain from the past is just below the surface, and what they are really saying to me is "This still hurts, and I'm scared to go there. *I'm scared to be vulnerable.*" So, what happens instead is that we run and/or try to numb ourselves.

Now, this is the bit I want you to pay close attention to. Running away from or numbing past hurts is actually harder and more painful than facing them and processing them. It's not the past events that matter as much as the *meaning* we gave to those past events. The events that happened to us in the past fundamentally shape our present and future. There is no avoiding this; we have all been shaped/programmed in this way because, for whatever reason, we don't have the skills to reframe past events, particularly traumatic ones.

Many of us have experienced some form of trauma, either large or small. Trauma, or abuse of some kind, can be a life-altering event, and I will discuss this later in this chapter. What I want to explore first is the experience of trauma in more minor events, as this is a universal experience. These events could include anything from the kids who ignored or bullied you in school to your dog dying or someone making a rude thoughtless comment that stunned you.

What often makes these experiences traumatic is that our feelings around them weren't permitted or processed but were buried instead. Ascribing meaning to these events forms the idea of who we are in our minds and what our place is in the world. We often do this in an unhelpful way by forming beliefs about ourselves that limit us—you are not being included because there's something wrong with you, no one cares about the pain of losing your dog, your feelings don't matter, and so forth. We interpret past events subjectively, give them meaning and create a limiting belief based on this applied meaning (which is based on perception, not necessarily reality), and bury it in our subconscious mind. Because these feelings remain unprocessed we then relate current events back to these past ones. We will be taking a deeper dive into what limiting beliefs are and how they sabotage your sobriety in the "Pillar of Growth" chapter.

Journal Prompts to Start Process Work

How do you feel when you reflect on your past?
> Example: *I feel a knot in my stomach as there are some things that I think about that still make me feel uncomfortable. I know I have been avoiding them for years, and it's gotten me nowhere.*

Do you feel that these unresolved events have affected you?
> Example: *I think they have. I am beginning to see how I always expect to be let down. I don't want to, but when someone lets me down I feel it's inevitable. I want to understand why this keeps happening to me, and how I can change it.*

What would be the first step to healing this?
> Example: *I think I could take a risk and talk to someone about it.*

...

THE SUBCONSCIOUS MIND

Understanding how the conscious mind and subconscious mind work will be very helpful to your growth, and I will be referring to the subconscious mind a lot in this and the next chapter.

Our conscious mind is the part we are aware of. It's where our thoughts are, and it's interested in the here and now. We think the conscious mind is big because we are aware of it, but it's not anywhere near as big as the subconscious mind, which we are not aware of. The conscious mind is responsible for about 5 percent of what happens in our life, which means the subconscious mind is responsible for a whopping 95 percent of what happens to us.[1] This has major implications for our sobriety.

Many things start in the conscious mind and then move to the subconscious mind. The reason for this is that it's more energy efficient. Once something has been learned or a meaning about an event has been created unchallenged, it moves to the subconscious mind. How we learn to drive a car is a good example of this. We have to do it very consciously at first and bring our awareness to what we are doing, but eventually the "how to" part goes into our subconscious mind, and we don't think about how to drive, we just do it. The subconscious mind is absorbing information and data all the time about what it means to be us and creating programs so our responses are automatic, meaning we don't have to think about how to respond, we just do.

An automatic programmed response learned through years of driving can come in handy if a car swerves in front of us, but an auto response that stems from a past event totally unrelated to a present one . . . not so much. For example, if we had a parent who shouted at us a lot when we were kids, and we felt that this was our fault and therefore felt shame, then this belief and the feelings associated with it get buried in our subconscious. So, thirty years later when our boss shouts at us, we don't think,

That's completely unacceptable, we instead get flooded with feelings of shame and start thinking that our boss shouting at us must be our fault. Our subconscious mind tells our conscious mind that this *present thing* is like this *past thing*, and therefore you must feel this preprogrammed way. It's an auto response.

Our reaction to the present event is automatic and based on past events, and all this information is buried in our subconscious mind. We are subconsciously responding to a *cue*. And our response to that cue will be determined by the past until we know differently and can change it. Which is why we all must understand how the past has shaped our present.

We will find that we have these automatic predetermined reactions before we are really even aware of it. What makes this reaction so powerful is that we experience the subconscious mind's response in our bodies. The body will take over and be in control. Our emotions, not our rational brain, are running the show. When our parent shouted at us as a kid, our bodies would have been flooded with emotions; we would have felt the *sensations* of shame, fear, abandonment, and so forth. It's from these types of experiences that we form and reinforce limiting beliefs about ourselves.

Limiting beliefs are how we give meaning to events so we can catalogue them. They are then stored in our subconscious mind where they shape our lives. This is another reason willpower doesn't work, as this physical experience and our limiting beliefs are way more powerful than willpower. Remember I've been saying all through this book that we drink because of how we feel. If we are flooded with these feelings and have no idea how to change or manage them, then alcohol will provide handy relief. Understanding and changing this is the deeper work of sobriety.

I want you to understand that the subconscious mind works like your computer hard drive—it operates according to how it is programmed. The conscious mind is the computer keyboard. It really doesn't matter how hard we pound the keys—if the programming is faulty, our computer won't do what we want it to do. So, if we want the computer to be more effective, we have to change the programming. Once we understand this, we can set about fixing it. Uncovering this faulty programming and changing it will not just have a revolutionary effect on your sobriety but on your entire life as well. Process and growth work are very much about reprogramming our subconscious thinking.

THERE WAS SOMETHING WRONG WITH ME

One of the fundamental limiting beliefs I formed about myself was that there was something wrong with me. When we are young and not given any support to manage our emotions, our negative experiences and the *meaning* we give to them will be absorbed and transferred to our subconscious minds without protest. Through my work as a therapist I have come to realize that the belief of not being good enough and that something is wrong with you is unbelievably common. We all have wildly different experiences but still come up with the similar limiting beliefs. Why is that?

I believe it goes back to not being taught how to deal with our feelings or emotions. The lack of emotional literacy in our culture means that so many of us struggle to process what we experience in a healthy way, but if we are unable to do so, it gets pushed down or ignored. We then reexperience these beliefs as feelings when they are triggered by present events. Something happens and our brains go, *This is like the time when all the girls in my class ignored me for a whole day* and then *boom* your subconscious mind brings forth the uncomfortable feeling that went with the *past* event and links it to the present one. This feeling is hard to ignore and very unpleasant. Who wouldn't want to change it? I know I did, and I know alcohol was my go-to, so I didn't have to experience how awful I felt about myself.

Here's an example. I was dating this guy for a few weeks, and I really thought he was "the one." I had started an affair with him while I was engaged to someone else, and I left my fiancé for him, but not long after our relationship started, I could feel him leaving me. Panicked and terrified of being alone, I did everything I could to hold on. Then came the phone call, and he said it was over. The feeling of abandonment that hit me was intolerable—my worst fears were confirmed: *This is like when my dad walked out on me—there must be something wrong with me that keeps this happening. I'm just not good enough.* And I ran to the liquor store and bought two bottles of wine because I couldn't tolerate how it felt to be me. I couldn't be in my head, and I had no tools for dealing with these feelings, so I chose to numb.

What I was doing was telling myself a story over and over that there was something wrong with me, and I wasn't good enough. It became a program, a script, a pattern that just kept running, and I would only see things that reinforced it. When I got sober, I realized I couldn't outrun myself any longer and that I had to understand why I kept producing results in my life that I didn't want. I had to begin to understand why I felt and reacted the way I did, why I had these patterns. I had to start the process of healing.

All of the pillars work together, and process and growth are very closely linked because process work automatically results in growth. And growth can often lead to more process (understanding). Once we understand what the process of growth is and what happens, we can more effectively overcome our limiting beliefs.

PROCESSING THE PAST

Dealing with your past, and to be really accurate, with your programming that *originated* from your past, is some of the most important work you will ever do. It's never too late to start or too early to begin. The most lethal assumption we can make is to believe that *this is just how it is* or *it's too late*. We believe we can't change things or that we can't change our thinking or our outcomes. These are all limiting beliefs, but we are not faulty or broken—we were just programmed incorrectly. It's not fair or right; it just is. It's up to us to choose what to do from there.

When we undertake the work of understanding how our past shapes our present, we can change unhelpful patterns (like drinking too much, overeating, overspending, and so forth) and grow into better versions of ourselves. When we become free of its "hooks" and change the faulty programming, then the past transforms into *wisdom*. This is an extremely valuable asset to have. We can't change the past, but we can change how we feel about it.

If we are really going to boil this down, the essence of process work is to examine and change the meaning we give to past events. It is the meaning we created that we carried forth into our future. And this is how our past is *controlling* our present experience.

Because I believed there was something wrong with me, I kept creating events and circumstances that *reaffirmed* that belief. The outcome was already set. This was done in my subconscious mind. I had already absorbed the message that there was something wrong with me, so my mind followed that program and created circumstances that kept reinforcing it. Once I uprooted that faulty thinking and transformed the meaning I had assigned to these past events, it had an immediate impact on my life.

Some of us have unresolved issues from the past. This can be in the form of trauma, hurt, injustice, or abuse of various kinds that lie like untreated wounds just below the skin—they only need a little bump to be opened up again. Many people carry them for their whole lives. These wounds won't heal on their own. They need to be in the light of day—cared for, honored, and healed.

We don't want to be "owned" by the past; we want to integrate those events, so they are just part of the rich tapestry of our lives. This is key: we get to choose our response to those events, no matter how painful they were.

Our past "owns" the present when we keep triggering the feelings and emotions and reliving the experience. Limited by the beliefs and meanings we formed, our past blocks us and prevents us from growing or moving forward and from reaching our potential and embarking on becoming the person we were meant to be. This is why process work is such an important pillar of sustainable sobriety.

THE RELATIONSHIP PROCESS

One of the most common ways our past shows up in our present is in our relationships with others. How we relate to others is something we usually learn in childhood. We all have patterns in our friendships, in our families, and, in particular, in our romantic relationships.

Perhaps we feel distrustful of others: we expect them to let us down or hurt us. Or we feel it is our responsibility to make our partner happy, that our feelings are secondary. Maybe relationships are hard for you, and you always feel left, rejected, or alone. All of these are examples of your past showing up in your present. How we relate to others, what we expect to happen, the feelings that we have when we get close to people—all of those experiences were learned when we were young. Most of us experience some kind of difficulty in our dealings with other people. I often hear my clients say, "This always happens to me. I always get let down" or "I just give and give, but I never feel good enough." This is a pattern. If we want to change it, we need to go through the process of uncovering where it came from.

One way to start on process work is to understand our attachment style in relationships. Our attachment style shows up in all our relationships, but particularly in romantic ones. We *all* have patterns in romantic relationships. These come from early childhood programming in our families, where we learned to deal with our feelings by what was modeled around us. It's often hard to spot these patterns in ourselves, which is why we repeat them with different partners. It really doesn't matter who shows up—we will subconsciously start acting out our attachment needs in the relationship.

Attachment

The concept of attachment has been well researched and documented over the past few decades. We now know that infant attachment is crucial for the well-being of children. Just like they need food, milk, warmth, and safety, they need to feel that their needs are also going to be met by their primary caregiver. Attachment is when a child feels like their big person loves them and is going to meet their needs. Numerous mental, emotional, and physical issues arise if an infant's attachment needs aren't met. These issues can affect them for the rest of their lives. Being able to form connections with others is fundamental to our well-being and happiness. How we attach to others is a behavior that plays out throughout our adulthood.

In Amir Levine and Rachel Heller's book *Attached*, the writers outline the following three attachment styles:

- Anxious (worry that their partners will leave them)
- Avoidant (don't want their partners to get too close)
- Secure (are comfortable with vulnerability and available for intimacy)[2]

These styles of attachment originate in childhood and then manifest themselves in our adult romantic relationships. They shape how we respond to intimacy, whether we allow ourselves to be vulnerable, and whether or not we can sustain long-term romantic attachments and friendships.

The key word here is intimacy. Intimacy is a meaningful connection. Remember when we explored this in the chapter on connection? There is only one path to meaningful connection and that is through vulnerability. How we approach vulnerability will be dictated by our attachment style.

In my past relationships, I was anxiously attached. The fear of being left or abandoned was always just below the surface, and the slightest thing could trigger it. I can trace this back to an emotionally unavailable father and mother. Interestingly, I always managed to attract avoidant personalities. Avoidants want intimacy and connection—it just really scares them, so as soon as they start getting close to someone they have to start pulling away. It is also possible to be a combination of the two. I have also felt avoidant of people when vulnerability just felt too risky.

We know that we all need and want meaningful connection; however, we continue to recreate situations in our lives where we are unable to receive it, or we push it away.

What Is Secure Attachment?

Secure attachment is when we can feel comfortable with intimacy and can feel safe enough to be vulnerable. Someone who is securely attached has good boundaries and is able to communicate their needs and feelings appropriately.

When you are securely attached, you don't need your partner to save you. You have saved yourself. You want an equal partnership, can tolerate your partner having their own space away from you without feeling distressed, and feel safe to open up to them as the relationship progresses. Secure attachment in a relationship comes from a secure relationship with ourselves. And we can only feel secure in ourselves when we understand our patterns and heal our hurts.

Original Pain

I had a very well-established pattern in my relationships with men. Men were dazzled by me. They thought I was amazing. I felt magical under their gaze. My relationships would get very intense very quickly (pheromones!), and I would feel like I was in love and this was it. This was "the one." I was sure that forever more we would live in this bubble of bliss and mutual adoration. Love was the answer.

And then *it* would happen. Every time, without fail.

I would notice a very subtle shift, almost invisible to the naked eye, but I would *know*. It was the beginning of the pulling away. Panic and terror would ignite within me, and I would move to a vigilant state. I was prepared to go to any length, take any action, to prevent the object of my love from leaving me.

I never could prevent it. They always left. All of a sudden, the adoration they used to pour on me would begin to leak away. They did not want to spend every moment with me. They were not thinking of me every second of every day. They were leaving our perfect bubble and going back to the world. And I felt like I was going to die. I would try very hard to get them to stay. I would tie myself up in knots trying to be thinner, prettier, funnier, smarter, or whatever I felt it was they wanted. I would be accommodating, pleasing, understanding (oh, so understanding). I would gladly accept the crumbs from the table they were now giving me. I welcomed any scrap of attention (usually sexual) until they finally pried off my fingers and made a hasty exit—leaving me in a black hole of despair.

The aloneness that hit me after felt like drowning. Alone . . . I was always alone. Not good enough, not worthy of love. Broken, with no idea of how I was going to get through the rest of my days without them. Somehow, I would piece myself back together. I would try to quell the frantic anxiety within. And then, after a bit of time, I would start it all over again with someone else—with the same results.

When I was going through this, I thought it was because I hadn't found "the one." If only I could find them then all would be well. But this isn't true. It's not about finding "the one." It's about *becoming* "the one."

The pain we feel when a romantic relationship ends is original pain. Only part of it is related to the actual relationship. The rest is unprocessed pain from our childhood. The original pain I felt came from my father's abandonment of me when I was five years old. Deep down I always felt like I was going to be left.

Most of us don't get very good lessons on how to deal with our feelings, so we just stuff those feelings down inside. They don't go anywhere, they just sit in the storage container, waiting. Sometimes they try to get our attention, but we have developed many quick fixes, so we don't have to deal with them, fixes like drinking alcohol, overeating, scrolling on our phones. This is the pain we carry around from childhood, and it will be triggered in our romantic relationships. When we feel like we are being left, abandoned, or ignored, our brains say, *This feeling is just like this other feeling* (we have been carrying around), and it joins the two together. So, the unbearable pain you experience when a relationship fractures or breaks is only partly due to that specific event. What your brain is doing is accessing *original* pain. That's why it cuts so deeply.

If we have ever experienced this more than once (generally we repeat patterns in relationships), then we must process the past so that if we are anxiously attached, we can begin to feel less panic if someone doesn't want to spend all their time with us. Or if we are avoidant, we can feel less frightened by opening up and becoming vulnerable. It's only by healing the hurt from the past and interpreting these events differently that we can get free. This is why we need to process the past.

How Alcohol Affects Our Relationships

Alcohol and romance are very much entwined. Alcohol is marketed in such a way as to suggest that using alcohol leads to romantic success (and sex). When we use alcohol appropriately, it is merely a small addition; it should never be the main fuel. Yet for many of us, alcohol is a significant and often destructive factor in our romantic relationships.

Think back on your romantic relationships and the part alcohol played in them. I know that for me, alcohol was the only way I could have a relationship (let alone have sex!). It made me feel safe enough to feel I could risk intimacy. Relationships, sex, and intimacy are all built on a foundation of vulnerability, and if you can't be vulnerable then you need something to assist you, so you at least have a façade of vulnerability. I used alcohol to hide the real me and project a fake version of myself, so that I felt comfortable enough to be close to someone and get the connection I craved.

Relationships can be scary, and we often feel like we need a crutch. Alcohol provides a false feeling of safety and comfort that we use to establish a romantic attachment. As we have discussed, alcohol is marketed to us as a vehicle for experiencing all the feelings we crave. It is certainly marketed as a way to experience intimacy and sex, as well as connection and belonging. These are linchpins to a romantic relationship; they are the structure that holds it up. Apart from the pheromones that are triggered when we are sexually attracted to someone, we also feel a sense of belonging—we feel that this person really gets us, knows us from the inside out. These feelings are intoxicating. Of course, many happy and functioning romantic relationships include alcohol, but the reason these are sustainable is that alcohol is not a central feature or the glue that binds people together. It's not used as a method to mask vulnerability.

When you feel ready, take a hard look at how alcohol has affected your relationships. What part did alcohol play? I have many clients who married their drinking buddy. Alcohol was a key and dominant part of their relationship. All socializing and celebrating required alcohol use. When it became clear to one of the partners that alcohol was indeed a problem, there was also a lot of fear about what would happen if they stopped drinking—how would the relationship function?

This is one of the saddest things for me to see. I have many clients who want to get sober but are scared to because their whole relationship is built around alcohol use. It is certainly more challenging to stop drinking when one's partner is unsupportive or is even sabotaging their efforts by drinking. Will the relationship survive? Maybe, maybe not. But I do know that if you don't save yourself then there will be nothing left of the relationship anyway. If you are in this situation it is crucial to get expert support, as this is too hard a road to navigate alone. Some clients worry about whether they have anything else in common with their partner or wonder what they will even do together if they aren't drinking. Alcohol can fill up a lot of cracks.

Whether you are single, dating someone, married, or celibate, understanding how you show up in your romantic relationships is a key part of process work. Because it is so linked to patterns from our family of origin, it is often one of the first areas of work I undertake with a new client. You can't really work on one without examining the other.

Suggestions for Understanding
Your Relationship Patterns

Nearly everyone struggles with relationships, and there are lots of things you can do if you have recognized yourself in this chapter. Certainly information is key. Check the resources section at the back of this book for a list of helpful books. Investing in work with a therapist or relationship coach would also be of benefit, and I would suggest writing a history of your romantic relationships to look for patterns in your behavior.

Journal Prompts to Understand Attachment and Relationships

What attachment style do you identify with?

Example: *Avoidant. I get anxious if people start getting close and push them away and make excuses.*

How has this affected your relationships and friendships?

Example: *I can see a pattern now and how I feel lonely yet don't let people in.*

What deeper work are you discovering?

Example: *I can see how my childhood has affected me.*

Describe your ideal relationship.

Example: *One that is based on respect. I want to be seen. I want to feel like an equal.*

...

UNCOVER, DISCOVER, DISCARD

Process work is a journey. It is like peeling an onion—it can make you cry, and there are always more layers. But the journey and the layers are crucial, as that is how we learn. I often hear it said that life doesn't come with an operating manual. It actually does and it's inside us, buried and waiting to be found. It's the authentic connection to our feelings and emotions. Generally, when we find our operating instructions, they are faulty. There are a lot of unhelpful programs that are running and producing results we don't want. However—and this is the good news—we can fix the parts that aren't working effectively so that we can operate as secure, grounded, balanced people—and get different results.

Process work always follows a pattern: uncover, discover, discard.

The uncovering process is when we begin to go below the surface and pull this stuff out for the first time. Most of us don't know it's there. This is what you're doing right now, holding this book. You are uncovering things about yourself that you never knew were there.

The next stage is to discover. Discover what this means, where it comes from, why we have felt this way, why we have avoided it for so long. The discovery stage in many ways can last our whole lives, as long as we remain curious about ourselves.

We can also discard. When I begin to understand that the voice in my head saying, *There's something wrong with you* is not an all-knowing truth but simply a belief I picked from interpretation of childhood events, then I have the keys to my freedom. I can dismantle and challenge that voice, refuse to act on it, and eventually replace it with *You are worthy*. We can discard the past programming that no longer serves us.

Journal Prompts to Begin the Process of Uncover, Discover, Discard

What have you uncovered about yourself from reading this book so far?

Example: *Until now, I really didn't see the link to my childhood and how I people please. I've always felt anxious about needing to fit in and be accepted by my peers. I thought it was just the way I was.*

What have you learned from these discoveries?

Example: *I am beginning to see that there is a real link between how I feel and how I act. I can sometimes act rashly and then regret it. Now I am seeing that it's how I try to get rid of uncomfortable feelings.*

What are you ready to discard?

Example: *I don't want to be the kind of person who drinks just because her friends do. I want to behave in ways that mean I like myself regardless of what others think. I want to let go of that behavior.*

...

TRAUMA

The question is never "Why the addiction?" but "Why the pain?"

DR. GABOR MATÉ[3]

I cannot emphasize enough how important it is to be trauma-informed in our recovery from an alcohol problem. So many of us have buried trauma in our past. There are many behaviors that are related to managing trauma: food disorders, alcohol and drug abuse, and workaholism, to name just a few. So many of us are carrying emotional pain that shows up in our behavior. When we understand this perspective it makes sense, and our response can be so much more informed. Trauma is a public health crisis and addiction is the front line. Culturally, we are not very good at dealing with feelings, especially extreme feelings, so our trauma remains unprocessed, unseen, and trapped within us. Our buried feelings related to our trauma are begging us every day to be seen, validated, and learned from.

We have discussed how many of us can experience trauma in minor events. I now want to explore trauma as a life-altering event. Trauma can be understood as a one-time experience (like a car accident) or an ongoing experience (like sexual abuse). There is no hierarchy of trauma—any degree of trauma can have a devastating effect on someone's life, as discussed. However, there is a difference when the trauma is an event that is a threat to life or a *perceived* threat to life.

One of the most groundbreaking pieces of research is the Adverse Childhood Experiences (ACEs) study on the impact of childhood trauma.[4] This study has shown the link between traumatic episodes experienced as a child and the propensity for not just addiction but for multiple physical and mental health problems in adulthood. It seems obvious now; however, I feel that for many years we have had this belief that there is some sort of magic that occurs when one becomes an adult—that regardless of your childhood experiences, when you become an adult, you should just get over it and get on with it; you should know the difference between right and wrong and should conform to society's expectations of you. "Push your feelings down, as they do not matter" is the message we have been given.

I am certainly not excusing criminal or harmful behavior by someone who is suffering from an addiction. There need to be consequences and restitution for those actions. However, when you have experienced trauma as a child, knowing right from wrong is irrelevant. What you are dealing with is pain or no pain. All of your actions stem from trying to manage internal emotional chaos. Because of how trauma affects our brains, trauma will replay itself over and over no matter how many years have gone by. When someone feels this way, all they are doing is responding to how they feel (pain or no pain). Their historical trauma is triggering physical and emotional reactions that they have little control over in the moment because their brain chemistry has changed.

As Bessel van der Kolk says in *The Body Keeps the Score*, "After trauma the world is experienced with a different nervous system. The survivor's energy now becomes focused on suppressing inner chaos at the expense of spontaneous involvement in their life."[5] I want to put this in really relatable terms. Internal emotional pain and chaos feel very similar to physical pain. If you can recall the worst physical pain you have ever been in (for me it was childbirth), you know that all rational thoughts go out the window, and all you want to do is to make the pain stop by any means. It is irrelevant what those means are—legal or illegal, moral or immoral, honest and "good" or not—the need to stop the pain overrules everything else.

Emotional pain (the wound just below the surface) is exactly the same. Not everyone who has experienced some kind of childhood trauma ends up on drugs or abusing alcohol, of course. However, what we now know is that they could graduate from college, become an esteemed professional, and on the outside look like an outstanding citizen. But on the inside, they can be plagued with depression, obsessive-compulsive disorder, anxiety, or low self-esteem; it's just hidden. That is what is so astounding about the ACEs research. It has revealed that children who experience trauma have a much higher risk of developing heart disease, cancer, stroke, bronchitis, emphysema, diabetes, hepatitis, jaundice, and skeletal fractures.[6]

Before, we just thought many of these conditions were the luck of the draw. Of course, some lifestyle issues and genetic predispositions are also at play, but we now know there is a clear and distinct link between the trauma we experience as children and the physical health challenges we may face as an adult.[7]

Bessel van der Kolk's *The Body Keeps the Score* brings together the research that supports the relationship between trauma and our physiology.[8] Traumatic experiences rewire our brain circuitry. Someone who has experienced trauma will not be capable of appropriate responses to certain events because their brains are wired in a different way. This was done initially as a coping mechanism: a traumatic event is overwhelming to our system, and the brain has to find a way to cope with it. We then get stuck in a pattern that is no longer helpful once the traumatic event has passed.

It is the same with our physiology. The mind and body are inextricably linked, and we experience our emotions as physical sensations in our bodies. One thing I say to my clients all the time is, "Check in with your body." Our bodies know how we are feeling, and they can't lie to us. Our bodies hold our trauma, but they also hold the key to our healing.

In his book *Waking the Tiger*, Peter A. Levine assures us that trauma is not a life sentence and with the right approach we can heal these wounds. He reaffirms that the key to healing is in our bodies as that is where the trauma is stored.[9] He also says, "The healing of trauma is a natural process that can be accessed through an inner awareness of the body. It does not require years of psychological therapy, or that memories be repeatedly dredged up and expunged from the unconscious."[10]

I find this assertion to be very hopeful. What he is saying is that it's not necessary to remember and record every detail of a past trauma, that healing can occur by connecting to the body and using appropriate therapeutic processes. He goes on to say that we retain traumatic symptoms because our reactions to traumatic events are incomplete. We haven't been allowed them or helped with them. And so we remain symptomatic until our trauma process is completed, and this can be done any time. I see so much of my clients' behavior through a trauma lens; indeed, I see it in most of our culture. If we put trauma-informed care at the front of our addiction and health services as well as in our culture, then we could change so much in this world.

This is why the ACEs research has the potential to change everything. I am a firm believer that if we do everything we can to minimize childhood trauma and become responsive to trauma in our communities, we will solve the majority of the world's problems.

WHEN TO START

It's really important to start when you feel ready and secure. I would strongly discourage you from opening up childhood trauma in the early days of your sobriety. Process takes time, and in order to start it, we must feel some degree of safety first and build a firm sober foundation. When you feel you have a foundation and support then it might be the right time to start. If you are engaged in a process of personal discovery, then it is inevitable that the work you need to do will come knocking at your door. Our job is to hear the knock and be receptive to the work.

We have been provided with incredible resources, many of them free. Make use of all the resources that are available to you in your community and online. A really effective way to start is trauma-informed yoga. No words, just movement. I think this is a really gentle and kind way to get connected with yourself and your body to begin the process of healing. I also recommend using Emotional Freedom Technique (EFT)—more about this later—and Eye Movement Desensitization and Reprocessing (EMDR) as effective tools for dealing with past trauma. Also search for sober-support services in your area, but make sure they are "trauma informed," which just means that they can recognize trauma responses and refer you to an appropriate professional. If you are fortunate enough to be able to pay for professional support, then invest in that also. There is nothing more valuable than our emotional well-being, so it's always worth the investment of time and money. If funds are limited there are many charities and low-cost options that may be available. Seek them out. There is a list of free resources and programs at the back of the book.

Learning to trust the process you are in is a key part of this work. We are always in a process of understanding, learning, and growing, and integrating that knowledge into our conscious and subconscious minds. Sometimes process work feels like driving in the fog. You know there is a road up ahead, but you can't see it—your headlights are only showing you ten feet ahead. So, we slow down, but we keep going because we know the rest of the road will appear. Even if we can't see it, we trust it will appear. Process work is a bit like that. We often can't see the road ahead, but that doesn't mean it's not there. Yes, it will feel scary at times—driving into the fog can often feel like that. But the road is taking you somewhere. It's a journey, and the things you see and learn on the journey don't just make it worthwhile, they allow you to change and grow.

OUR EMOTIONAL GUIDANCE SYSTEM

The reason we want to process our past is that if we don't, it blocks us from fully engaging with our emotional guidance system. Our emotional guidance system is our instructional manual for where we want to go. When we are fully connected to our bodies and can identify our emotions, we can use them to guide us. The five pillars are how we become connected to this internal guidance system. Just like the navigation system pilots have to help them fly to where they want to go, our emotions and feelings are a guidance system that will help us navigate our journeys. If a pilot ignored all their navigation equipment and instead just took off and flew in the direction they thought Brazil was in, they might feel a little bit angry and confused when they landed in Africa instead. They thought they knew the direction, but because they didn't listen to their navigation system, they went off course and ended up somewhere completely different. That's just what it's like trying to live without using our own internal navigation system. We just won't end up in the place we hoped to.

Our emotions and feelings are a particular kind of language that a lot of us just don't speak. Often, that's because it was never spoken in our family of origin. As I mentioned earlier, my family of origin had no emotional literacy. Dealing with our feelings and emotions in a healthy way was not talked about or modeled in any way. Feelings were shut down with looks and comments, so they became something quite scary for me. Because I didn't understand them, they frightened me and I buried them—stuffed them deep inside and poured alcohol on top of them to keep them quiet.

Maybe you did the same thing? Learning how to use my emotional guidance system was something I had to learn as an adult, and you can too. You are taking your first steps toward learning how to use your emotional guidance system by reading this book. The five pillars are designed to help you become attuned to your guidance system. When you are connected to your body, cultivate boundaries and balance, know how to meet your needs in a healthy way, and recognize past patterns and how you sabotage yourself, then you are using your emotional guidance system.

THE STORAGE CONTAINER

Because some of us have bottled up our feelings for so long and have never learned appropriate methods for dealing with our feelings, when we first get sober our emotions can often come out sideways in ways we don't understand.

I have used the term *storage container* throughout this book as a way to picture what we do with our feelings, and I want to explain in more detail what I mean by that. Imagine there is a storage container inside you, and every time something happens and you feel sad, frustrated, angry, disappointed, annoyed, scared, and so forth, you stuff those feelings into the storage container and secure the lid firmly. Now, we only do this with feelings that are difficult. We don't tend to want to run away from joy, happiness, or excitement, though we can sometimes feel unworthy of those feelings.

We continue to put the difficult feelings in storage, stuffing them down and neglecting to deal with them or learn from them, and we use various methods to ignore how we feel. Now, those feelings will demand your attention regularly. If you listen, you can hear them knocking on the door to be let out. *Absolutely not*, we think to ourselves, and we just find more things to stuff on top. Food, drugs, sex, shopping, scrolling on our phones—all of these activities can numb away the urgency of our feelings.

And then we get sober.

When we get sober, we can't keep a lid on our feelings anymore. The lid will open and they will begin to spill out. They will demand to be heard, to be seen, to be validated, and to be released. This can feel overwhelming and a little bit scary. I've often heard it described as a roller coaster. In the early days of sobriety this is why connection and support are so vital.

My father passed away from cancer when I was eighteen. I remember my mother calling me with the news, and I felt nothing—just numb, and it wasn't an "in shock" kind of numbness. I knew you were supposed to feel something when your father died, but I just couldn't access it. I faked my response because I could tell from the people around me that I needed to have some kind of reaction.

When I was about two years sober (eleven years after my father passed away) I came home from work one day and just felt overwhelmingly sad. I cried and cried. And this went on for days. I didn't try to fight it because it felt like relief. After a while I realized that it was a feeling of intense grief for my dad. I wrote him a letter, talked about him, and just felt all the feelings that you need to feel when you lose someone you love. All of these feelings had been in storage—waiting to come out, waiting until it was safe and I was able to handle them. And when everything subsided, I felt all the better for it; something inside of me had shifted.

No one wishes to be sad or to grieve, but we can't avoid these experiences if we want to have the fullest human experience we can possibly have. As Brené Brown says (and I paraphrase here), we can't selectively numb our feelings. We can't numb the bad and keep the good.[11]

The feelings of grief when we lose someone or something we care about are *necessary*. They are a necessary process that we have to go through and complete, otherwise these feelings get stuck inside us, and we can't grow. This is why growth and process are so linked. If we don't learn to process through our emotional landscape, then we can't grow either. We are stuck in a holding pattern. Existing but not *being*.

The delayed grief process I felt for the loss of my father allowed me to feel closer to him. It was painful, yes, but it was also enriching. It helped me feel closer to other people too. Loss is a universal human experience that binds us together. It allowed me to feel empathy for others in a way I hadn't experienced before, and empathy is an essential human skill to have.

As I said, I was at least two years sober before I could get anywhere near these feelings. I didn't understand at first what was happening, but through journaling (an essential processing tool) it was revealed to me. The feelings eventually subsided, as they always will, and what I discovered was that I had a deeper connection and understanding of myself. This unprocessed grief had created a block inside me, and I was unable to connect to a deeper part of myself until it had been released.

We will explore why connecting to the deepest part of ourselves is essential in the chapter on growth. However, I do want to say that when we feel more fully aligned with ourselves and have cleared some of this stuff away, we are able to use our internal navigation systems much more effectively. Before, it was like trying to see what the buttons and dials were saying, but there was a bunch of old paperwork dumped on the panel obscuring our view. Once we clear that old stuff away it is much easier to tune in to our emotions and use them to guide us in our decisions and choices.

Journal Prompts to Understand Your Storage Container

What emotional baggage do you feel you have been carrying around?

> Example: *I feel the weight of my parents and how they treated me as a child. I still feel insecure from when I was bullied at school.*

How does it feel carrying this?

> Example: *Like a dead weight.*

What help is available to you?

> Example: *There are online groups I could attend regularly, and I know there are some local support services I could check out.*

...

GET INTO YOUR BODY

One of the first things I teach clients who feel blocked emotionally is to get into their bodies. We experience our feelings and emotions as physical sensations in our bodies. Our brains and our bodies communicate with each other. When we don't understand these physical sensations and they scare us, our brains will search for the fastest method possible to feel comfortable again. This is one of the reasons alcohol is so addictive: it provides a really fast, really effective, and really cheap method to escape from emotions we are not prepared to experience.

Getting sober means becoming emotionally literate. This in itself is a process of trial and error. I want you to start by bringing your awareness to your body and noticing how your emotions show up. Notice where in your body you might feel a heaviness, pressure, or tightness—that may be an emotional response. Try to name the emotion—just take a guess. Is it trying to tell you something? Breathe through the uncomfortable feeling.

Here is the good news: experiencing your emotions when they happen is far easier than running from them. You also need to know that you will survive your feelings, whatever they are. This is very important, as the idea that I wouldn't survive my feelings was a core belief of mine and the big reason I ran from them and numbed them. I just didn't feel like I could do it. I used to say over and over to myself, *I will survive this, I will survive this*. And it was true—I did. I learned very quickly that supporting myself through these feelings made the process of dealing with them infinitely easier.

Telling someone how I felt (someone who could understand and support me) was life changing for me. It took away the threat of not surviving the feeling. This is your first step in process work. Get into your body and notice your feelings. Observe yourself with curiosity, not judgment, and support yourself when it happens. This is a life skill, just like riding a bike. The more you do it, the easier it will get. One of the most effective tools I use for calming my nervous system and feeling connected to my body is "tapping," or EFT. It connects the emotions in our bodies to the thoughts that accompany them. I am a Level 2 EFT practitioner and have found it infinitely helpful for myself and my clients. EFT is gentle tapping on acupressure points while repeating certain phrases. You can see some examples of tapping on my YouTube channel (Veronica Valli). EFT is very soothing and will help you regulate your emotions. It can also help considerably with trauma and any difficult feelings you are struggling with.[12]

RESPONDING INSTEAD OF REACTING

When we are disconnected from our emotional guidance system (our feelings and emotions), we tend just to react to things. This is often referred to as a trigger.[13] An external stimulus sets off an intense feeling (and bodily sensation) inside us, and our thoughts travel down very established neural pathways to respond with a behavior to end, subdue, or change the feeling we didn't like.

Because we have established these patterns over many years, most of them are in our subconscious, which means we are not really giving much thought to what happens. The actions are automatic—they are what happens when we let our emotions control us instead of controlling our *response* to them. And when we do this, we are not free. How many times have you messed up plans or arrangements or sabotaged situations or relationships because you were reacting to intense emotions? There have been countless times when I sabotaged plans I had by drinking, and I was drinking because that was how I reacted to intense emotions. When we learn to process our feelings in a healthy way, we gain emotional mastery, which means we can respond to what happens rather than just react. This gives us so much more control over our lives, which become calmer and more manageable when we are not a slave to our emotional reactions.

PROCESS AS A MUSCLE WE CAN BUILD

The only way we get mastery over our feelings is through practice. Over time we can learn to interrupt the neural pathways that lead us to have reactions that hurt us. With experience, we can begin to recognize that we can respond in different ways, and we'll see that this can become automatic.

Here is something you can try to begin this process:

1. When you notice emotions building up, pause and take a deep breath.

2. Describe what is happening in your body.
   Example: *My stomach feels tight and my heart is racing.*

3. Have a guess at what these feelings are linked to.
   Example: *It was that flippant comment my partner made.*

4. Then ask yourself *What is the story I am telling myself about what happened?* This question is transformational as it helps us uncover the limiting beliefs/programming that we are actually having the emotional response to.
   Example: *When my partner made that off-the-cuff remark I started telling myself it was because he doesn't care.*

5. Ask yourself if the story you're telling yourself is true in these circumstances.
   Example: *No, I know they care; they tell me and show me. It was a thoughtless comment, but I am putting way too much meaning on this.*

6. Now check in with your body and notice how you feel.
   Example: *A lot calmer and maybe a bit silly for overreacting?*

RESENTMENTS

One of the most difficult feelings I have ever had to manage is a feeling of resentment. Resentment is a mixture of pride, selfishness, and displeasure, and it is an extremely unpleasant feeling to experience. Resentments toward people can rent a lot of space in our heads (and can lead to the "free pass to get drunk"

I mentioned before). They can preoccupy us. I know instantly when I feel resentful toward someone, as I start planning revenge or how I am going to "show them" for some perceived slight. This is an immature reaction that is based on pride (don't they know who I am?) and the story I am telling myself about what happened. Now, as soon as I recognize that this is happening, I know I have a choice in how long I tolerate it. As soon as I am able to, I write it down. I examine it from different angles, and it begins to loosen its hold on me.

It is through this process that I can identify that their behavior wasn't personal but a manifestation of how they were feeling that I then interpreted personally. I created a meaning about this event that was false, and then I reacted to them based on the meaning I had created. Other people's behavior (including what they say) is simply a reflection of their inner state, not mine. It doesn't mean anything about me. I just make it about me. Understanding this is revolutionary in that it can have a dramatic effect on how you view and respond to others. I took other people's behavior personally (that is the essence of resentment—it feels very personal to us), and that's why it is so hard to let go of. I now know from experience that I have the power to release this feeling as soon as I want to—I just need to take certain actions. Because I am an imperfect human, I will feel like this from time to time. But I have built up the muscle that allows me to consider before I just react. I can choose to respond in a way that is healthy, and I can learn from the experience.

LEARNING EMOTIONAL LITERACY: THE JOURNEY TO EMOTIONAL SOBRIETY

When I say there is more to stopping drinking than stopping drinking, what I'm talking about is the process work. When we cross over the line from socially acceptable drinking (however that is defined) to drinking that no longer makes sense, we are inevitably using alcohol as a tool to cope with our emotional lives. That's what's so powerful about it. It's quick, easy, and effective. When we quit alcohol, if we want all that's promised in a sober life, we need to work toward emotional sobriety. Very simply put, *emotional sobriety is when we have appropriate emotional responses to events.*

When we are not fully aligned with ourselves and are blocked by our emotions, we often have inappropriate emotional responses to events. I have talked about my previous issues with relationships. When a relationship concluded with my being rejected, I would fall down a black hole of suicidal despair. Typically, the whole relationship lasted a matter of weeks. When a relationship ends, it can be painful, there is no doubt. However, the intense feeling I am describing is an inappropriate emotional response to this kind of relationship. I would feel like this even if the relationship lasted only two weeks. The reason for that, as I explained before, is that the pain I felt was not entirely related to the current relationship; it was in fact the original pain of abandonment that I kept acting out in my romantic relationships. Feeling sad, confused, and despondent when a six-week relationship ended would be appropriate. Suicidal despair wouldn't be. I did this in many areas of my life—abandonment and rejection would often be a theme, and if I perceived it, I would have very intense emotional reactions to it. If you canceled your plans with me, I felt rejected, unworthy, and intensely sad (inappropriate). Now, however, I would feel disappointed (appropriate) but be able to move on and replan my day.

This is how our emotional guidance system was designed to work. It was designed to enable appropriate emotional responses to the events and circumstances around us. We use the information our feelings give us to learn things and to grow, equipping us to deal with the next event, and so forth. We reflect and respond rather than just react. If I felt sad, I could recognize it and support myself through it rather than run away. Talking to someone, journaling, going to a support group were all ways I supported my difficult feelings, and all of these things helped make it feel better. Once in a while I will have an intense emotional response to something quite minor and because that is not now typical, I know immediately that there is something deeper there for me to explore. I welcome that exploration because I know from experience that it will lead to a deeper understanding—to an "aha" moment that will help me grow. Growth is so rewarding and juicy for me. I know whatever I am going through will make me richer, and I can now fully embrace these experiences. That is what I want for you too.

I want to repeat what I stated at the start of this chapter: you matter. I want you to think of all these past events that shaped your future as parts of yourself trapped in time. Imagine yourself at age five, ten, fifteen—whatever age you were when these difficult events occurred. Picture that child or young person and feel compassion toward them. They matter too. And they are waiting for you to notice, to bring your time and attention to see them, heal them, love them, and ultimately free them. By not understanding our past, we are saying that young person doesn't matter. It's much easier to have compassion for a child, so I want you to picture yourself as a child. Just tell that image in your mind that you see them, they matter, and you are starting the journey to heal them.

Start it now.

Journal Prompts to Begin the Process Pillar

Now that you have read this chapter, how do you feel? Check in with your body.

> Example: *A bit churned up. I feel a heaviness in my chest. I am beginning to connect the dots between the stuff in the past and how I drink.*

How can you support yourself with these feelings?

> Example: *They actually don't scare me quite as much now that I understand them a little better.*

How have you used alcohol to numb your feelings?

> Example: *I am beginning to see that I often drink because of the story I am telling myself about something that happened and that the story is not really accurate.*

What are your next steps to heal your past?

> Example: *I'm going to talk to my best friend as she knows me best—I'm going to be honest with her. I'm also going to seek out a therapist.*

...

CHAPTER 9

The Pillar of Growth

There is a Universal Law of Life. If you look around, you will see it is undeniably true: we are either growing, or we are dying. Look at a plant or a tree; it is either growing or dying. Look at an animal; it is either growing (maturing) or dying. Look at a company or organization; it is either growing (improving, adapting) or dying. Look at a person; they are either growing (maturing, getting wiser) or they are dying (not growing, not learning, not getting wiser). Do you see? We have to grow, or we die. And if we grow, then we are going to encounter fear, because growing always means encountering new experiences, and new experiences can bring fear. We just can't avoid growing. Becoming more (growing) is our purpose and our destiny. Our challenge is to continue to grow while managing the fear.[1]

VERONICA VALLI, *Why You Drink and How to Stop*

This is the truth. We MUST grow into the person we were always meant to be. That is our purpose. But we can't do that when alcohol takes up too much of our lives. When we are full of booze, we can't be full of the good stuff. Growth comes from stepping out in the world, taking risks, embracing new challenges, following our dreams. It comes from facing fears . . . and walking through them. It comes from making mistakes and learning from them. To truly achieve sustainable sobriety, we have to grow in our hearts, minds, and souls. This is what we came here for. By just reading this book you declared to yourself that you want more. This is an act of growth; you are examining parts of yourself you haven't looked at before. This could be your first step into a whole new life—stronger, better, and alcohol-free.

THE TWO WORLDS

We live in two worlds: the external one and the internal one. The external world concerns itself only with how things appear to others. Drinking when it no longer makes sense keeps us in the external world. We live in the external world, but our true home, our bedrock, is the internal one. It is our internal world that matters and where the source of our contentment lives.

The external world is what we have, what we get, what our job is, who our peers are, what other people think of us, what we look like, and so on. The problem is that we think what is in the external world is what really *matters* and that everything in the external world is the sum of who we really are. And it isn't. Our internal world is a sacred space and where we truly exist. It's where our truest self resides, our awareness lives, and our spirit breathes.

It is a tragedy to live only in the external world and never really know your internal one. When we are drinking more than we want to, we sacrifice a significant amount of bandwidth to our relationship with alcohol. By this I mean we spend time thinking about drinking, thinking about not drinking, drinking, and recovering from drinking. This can take up 20, 30, or even 50 percent or more of our bandwidth. We may not be thinking of it all of the time, but it bothers us when we do. We know our relationship with alcohol isn't making sense anymore, but we still haven't realized we can quit without missing out on anything.

Our bandwidth is one of the most precious things we have. It's the space we have in our head to think thoughts, the energy it takes to live our lives, and the capacity we have to get things done. Think about the energy and time you have spent thinking, debating, and arguing with yourself about alcohol and whether to drink or not drink, trying to control your drinking, regretting drinking, swearing off drinking. Frankly, it's exhausting. And to what end? You do not have unlimited resources, and if this is how you are spending them, then you don't have the energy for the other stuff that life is calling you to do: the other opportunities, directions, and relationships that are more aligned to your true self.

Take a step back and look at how much space alcohol occupies in your life. Going back to my analogy on sandwiches, I would not get a lot done (and I wouldn't have gotten this book written) if I was spending all day thinking about what sandwich I was going to eat today, then worrying that maybe I had too many sandwiches yesterday and maybe I shouldn't have a sandwich today. But then I think, *I really want a sandwich, and it's not fair that I can't have one. Why can't I just have one sandwich?* Then I have the sandwich and I regret it, and I think, *All right, that's it. I'm not having any more sandwiches for the rest of the month.* Can you see how exhausting that is and also how pointless? It's just a sandwich—it doesn't mean anything. It's just a drink—it doesn't mean anything either, apart from the meaning that you have ascribed to it, what you believe about it, and what you think it represents in your life.

We have explored how marketing and culture have influenced how we think about alcohol. We have learned how we formed beliefs and meaning about events that then get buried in our subconscious minds. Part of our growth is about examining all our programming and rejecting what doesn't feel authentic. Our relationship with alcohol is very complicated. Throughout this book, I have shown you that we can't just stop drinking and expect everything to feel okay. We have deeply programmed beliefs about what we think alcohol brings to our lives, and it takes time to let go of those. But consider this: Has all the time and energy you have spent on alcohol been worth it? Did alcohol deliver? Or are you using alcohol to help you feel better, to cope with life? Did you find that the "help" alcohol gave you was short-lived?

Then ask yourself, *Is this how I want things to be for the next month, year, ten years? Constantly juggling alcohol and its consequences, while never having the energy or resources to step into the life I could have?*

It's very easy to get lost in the details of life and miss the main event. We get distracted and lost. We look for outside fixes to inside problems, and we think we have a "life" but really, it's just ticking off days. I want to invite you to stop ticking off days and to take the first step into the life that is waiting for you. A better life, where alcohol rents no space in your head and where you have the energy, time, and resources to grow into the person you were always meant to be.

THE CRITICAL VOICE/VOICE OF THE EGO

Before I walk you through the process of growth and how resistance shows up, I want to clarify how our ego voice, often referred to as the *critical voice* or *inner critic*, works. Dr. Nicole LePera, a holistic psychologist, explains this very well in her YouTube videos.[2]

Very simply, the ego tells us the story of who we *think* we are. The ego is not who you are. It's part of your identity and has a purpose. The primary purpose of the ego is to keep you safe. For example when you step too close to traffic, the voice shouts in your head, *Get back!* But it also does this in other situations, like when you have a new opportunity, maybe something out of your comfort zone. Perhaps this is something you have wanted for a while but when it actually happens you feel frightened. The ego voice may be saying things like, *Hold on there. What if this doesn't work out? What if you mess up? People will realize you are stupid! It might not work out and then you will have failed.* You may recognize some of these messages. The ego is just repeating the limiting beliefs that you have about yourself (the story of who it *thinks* you are).

In her book *5 Weeks to Self-Confidence* Lynn Matti describes the inner critic as "a devious little being who capitalizes on discomfort, fear, and stress. Your critical inner voice carries on a running, mostly subconscious monologue of judgment and personal attacks. It is most active when you want to take a risk or step outside your normal routine and comfort zone."[3]

When we listen to this voice, it sabotages us. And it is doing it because it wants to keep you in what is *familiar.* The ego doesn't want things to change. It wants to create a future that is similar to the past (which is why we have patterns and repeat the same mistakes). We are listening to this voice and making decisions based on what it is saying. Because most of us don't realize what is happening, we listen to this voice *all the time.* We cave in to it, we obey it, we let it govern our life. But remember that the ego is not who we are, we are not these stories it tells us about ourselves; rather, we are just recycling old beliefs about ourselves into our present. The ego is part of us, but it is not our authentic self. Most people don't know this, and the voice of the ego can be very powerful and *feel* like truth. I want you to know what is actually happening in your thoughts and how the ego is causing you to self-sabotage. Because the land of sobriety is unfamiliar and unknown, the ego will send you lots of messages about how it is unnecessary for you to go there. The critical voice will do whatever it needs to keep you in your comfort zone. But if we stay in what is comfortable, we can't grow.

THE DISCOMFORT OF GROWTH

I won't sugarcoat this. One of the reasons we avoid growth is that it's always uncomfortable, sometimes painful, and can take up a lot of energy. However, so does staying stuck. Not growing, avoiding it, running from it, repeating dysfunctional patterns over and over and getting the same results (the ones you don't want)—all of this takes up a lot of energy and is extremely uncomfortable. Choosing the discomfort of growth over the discomfort of staying stuck where you are is always worth it. I think we can forget as adults that we still need to grow, and that growth never ends. We are not "done" when we reach adulthood; in fact, we are really only beginning. We all know that childhood is all about growth—not just physically, but mentally, emotionally, and spiritually too.

Look at the effort kids put into growing. Right now, I have a son who is about to go into kindergarten. He has some fine-motor-skill issues, which means holding a pencil and writing his name requires some effort. He really has to concentrate on putting his fingers in the right place on the pencil and applying pressure in the right way so that he can form a letter. At some point we all went through this process, but then we mastered it, and it became a subconscious action. We don't think about holding a pencil now—it's a skill we grew into. And the process of learning to do it was uncomfortable until it wasn't.

That's basically how growth works. It's uncomfortable until it isn't. The discomfort is never a reason not to grow. In fact, learning to manage and sit with discomfort is a life skill we can learn if we choose to. As adults I think we have internalized a message that we should never have to feel uncomfortable. Of course, that's how marketing works. It persuades us that if we don't like how we feel, we can buy something that will give us feelings we desire, without much effort on our part. A quick fix. I want to bring this to your awareness and help you understand that discomfort is a good thing. I know it doesn't always feel that way, but if we allow ourselves the discomfort of growth, wonderful things can happen.

THE CALLING

We are all being called to grow—this is part of being human. Just as children are designed to explore, question, and test—constantly asking, "What's this?" "What does it do?" "Who am I?" "What does this mean?" This process was never designed to stop in childhood. We as adults are also being called to question, to wonder, to explore. This "calling" is a feeling deep inside you. Glennon Doyle, in her book *Untamed*, describes it as her "knowing."[4] But we often drift really far away from it because we get lost in the external world. The external world does not have the anchors that our internal one does, so we are unanchored, and we lose our way. We lose ourselves, and we lose our *knowing*, and we get lost in the details of our lives. And drinking alcohol is a detail—a really minor, minuscule detail. But somehow it can become the main event. Alcohol is an inanimate thing that our culture has ascribed meaning to, and we have internalized this meaning without question.

Growth is about reconnecting to the main event—*your main event*. The main event is your calling to grow into a purposeful, nourishing, and productive life. I have no idea what this would mean for you, but I *do* know there is something calling you. And you need at least to get onto the dance floor. I can tell you that your purpose is not sacrificing a percentage of your bandwidth by fighting with yourself about whether you are going to drink or not today. That is not what you came here to do.

The calling will feel very uncomfortable, because we have typically spent a long time not only ignoring it but actively moving away from it. The calling will feel frightening because it is new, uncharted territory. To listen to the calling, we have to be conscious and present—but most of all we have to get honest with ourselves about who we really want to be.

Alcohol often takes us away from who we want to be, and it is painful when we finally see that. But this is square one. Square one on the board is about acceptance—completely accepting that this is where we are. I can't move toward where I want to be without first accepting where I am. I know it doesn't feel great, but accepting where you are is actually easier than pushing against it, which is what you have been doing up to now. Fighting something is hard work. We need to start where we are. But this is not a goal-setting exercise; it's about accepting the fact that we are on the first square and looking for the next one.

Journal Prompts to Begin the Process of Uncovering Your Calling

How do you want to feel about yourself?

Example: *I want to feel comfortable in my own skin. I want to like myself. I want not to hurt or be scared anymore. I want to fulfill my potential. I want to feel free.*

What can you do now that will move you toward those feelings?

Example: *I can take this "not drinking" thing seriously. I can accept that alcohol is not a source of relief; it's a source of pain. I can start exercising a bit more and eating better. I can do some volunteer work, so I get out of the house and meet people. I can get some professional help to talk about the stuff that's been bothering me for years.*

What do you want to move toward?

Example: *I want to have an impactful life. I want to be of service to others. I want real friendships and a respectful life partner. I want to work in a career that I enjoy. I want to be fit and healthy.*

What are the details you keep getting lost in?
Example: *Drinking, thinking about drinking, being hungover, worrying what other people think, worrying about things I can't control.*

How are you being called?
Example: *I want to _____. I'd love to _____. I keep imagining myself as _____.*

How do you sabotage your calling?
Example: *I drink and it takes up too much time and energy. I talk myself out of things. Change feels scary so I put it off. Other peoples' opinions or reactions can divert me.*

Write out the answers and then observe what you feel. Notice any sadness, frustration, or feelings of regret. Also notice any resistance that comes up, especially if it's accompanied by that little voice in your head that is muttering lots of self-defeating and unhelpful comments. Writing these answers will probably feel a little uncomfortable. And that's great! That just means you're growing! I want you to pay attention to that niggle inside you. That is your calling; you have just awoken it, and it is going to be sending you messages. Take a deep breath and listen to what your calling is saying. This is square one. This is where your growth can start. Right now, today.

...

RESISTANCE TO GROWTH WILL SHOW UP

Dealing with resistance is an essential life skill, and I was well into my adulthood before I learned how to do it. It's so life-changing that it should be taught in schools (my children's school is teaching about mindset and mindfulness, so that's a good start). I spent years listening to the negative voice (the ego) in my head that was saying, *You can't do that. That won't work. Who do you think you are? You are going to fail so why bother?* I would get the call to growth and then resistance would kick in (as it always will), and I would buckle and retreat and not change or stretch myself. I believed the discomfort would end if I retreated, but all it did was delay it. I would go back to the place I was stuck in, where I didn't want to be, and try to convince myself it was okay. Then the call would come again, and I couldn't resist it so I would start moving, but I could never get through the discomfort. I just remained in this holding pattern, wanting to be more, but too scared to take the action.

If you pay attention to your thoughts, you will notice that the ego tells you the same story over and over regardless of what is happening in front of you. This is why we keep getting the same result. As author Eckhart Tolle says, "Most people are at the mercy of that voice; they are possessed by thought, by the mind. And since the mind is conditioned by the past, you are then forced to re-enact the past again and again."[5] So it's not the present circumstances that dictate the result, it's our *internalized beliefs* that do so. And the ego just repeats this back to us over and over. Then we get stuck in these familiar stories that aren't helpful and that stifle our growth.

The first step to dealing with that voice of resistance is to understand exactly what is happening. I am familiar with its pattern now. I have navigated around the ego many times. I expect it to show up as it always will, and I see it for what it is. The feeling of discomfort is still there, but because I know what is happening, it doesn't have mastery over me. I also feel a tinge of excitement as I know that I am growing into something, and this new thing

I'm growing into is going to help me expand and learn. There is a payoff, and I welcome the payoff of new awareness.

EGO SABOTAGE

Because of the ego voice and our mindset, we develop patterns of behavior that make us quite predictable. It doesn't matter the circumstances or person—we somehow produce the same result because it recreates feelings that are very familiar to us, feelings from our past. It is hard sometimes to see this in ourselves, but you may be able to spot patterns in people you know well. In fact, I bet there are a few people whose behavior you can predict very accurately. You know if X happens, they will respond with Y. Or if you say X, they will say Z. Or if Z happens, they will *feel* X.

The reason you know this is because you are familiar with their patterns and how they are programmed. They are predictable because the person's subconscious mind is in charge, as is yours, and this mindset is recreating feelings and outcomes that are familiar.

I am pointing this out as it's much easier to spot in other people, but rest assured, you do the exact same thing. You may think it's your circumstances that are creating your reality, but actually it's your beliefs *about* your circumstances that are creating your experience—which is why your behavior is just as predictable to other people as theirs is to you. Because the resistance the ego throws up feels so powerful, we fall into its trap and believe its messages, and we stay stuck. It feels authoritative and knowing, so we obey it until we know better. The voice of the ego can keep us small our whole lives, and it can also keep us drinking much longer than we need to be. We can experience revolutionary change in our lives when we undo the programming in our subconscious minds.

It's really important that you know this stuff because you are going to hear the call to grow when you stop drinking. In fact, I know you have been hearing the call even while you were drinking, otherwise you wouldn't be reading this book. There is just no avoiding the call to grow. Growth is about entering the unfamiliar, and that is always going to feel scary. And remember, the ego doesn't want you to leave the familiar so it will resist growth. It does not want you to grow—it likes things just as they are.

Many people experience this when they first think about quitting drinking. And it goes something like this: We drink, and one day we get *the calling*. This calling is your spirit, your inner self. It's the real you, and it's calling you to become your authentic self. When you feel that calling, your conscious mind will start thinking *That's it. I don't want to drink anymore. That was the worst hangover. I don't want this anymore. I hate feeling like I need to drink to fit in or have fun*. Then you will make a decision and begin to take some action. You will probably Google some stuff, order a book, listen to a podcast, and you will learn a bit more about sobriety and think, *Yeah, I can do this*.

Then you will start putting a few days of sobriety together and feel a bit better. Days turn into weeks and although some days are hard you are beginning at least to feel physically better. And then the voice of the ego will kick in, because it looks like you are dangerously close to leaving the land of alcohol and moving to the land of sobriety. You have never been to the land of sobriety before. Sure, you have stopped drinking for a few days or weeks, but nothing has really changed except that you have avoided situations where you might drink. But there is a vacation/holiday/birthday coming up, and you don't know how to navigate that without alcohol. The ego is sensing danger. It does not want you to move to the land of sobriety because that is unfamiliar, and the ego has no idea how to keep you safe there. It has lots of experience in the land of alcohol, however—it knows how to do that. The land of alcohol is familiar; it is the same thing over and over, and the ego can do it on autopilot.

And that's what the ego wants. It just wants familiarity. So, this is when you will start hearing the voice inside your head saying things like, *It wasn't that bad. Maybe you can just have one. Stick to wine and avoid spirits. Just drink on the weekends. Everyone else is having fun, why shouldn't you? You deserve it after the week you've had. Just this once won't hurt. You have a work event on Friday, and everyone will be drinking so maybe you can make an exception and just drink that night.*

These thoughts will be accompanied by uncomfortable feelings. You may feel churned up, angry, resentful, frightened, and all the uncomfortable feelings that no one wants to tolerate for too long. The voice of the ego is relentless, and it really kicks into high gear when our bodies start responding to its message. We experience our emotions in our bodies, and this particular uncomfortable feeling will be very fear based. The churning of the stomach, the tightness in our chest, the nervous energy—these physical experiences have been triggered by our thoughts. This creates a formidable combination. The ego will then step up and start presenting multiple ways for you to drink that seem very attractive. But most of all it is clearly signaling that all the discomfort in your body will go away *if* you listen to what the ego wants you to do.

You are *really* feeling the discomfort now, and the chatter is reaching a high volume. It is impossible to ignore, so you try to muster up the willpower to push through. All of your decisions and determination begin to crumble. You are fuzzy on why you wanted to stop drinking in the first place. Now sobriety feels hard, as you are actively working against yourself and trying to stay sober on willpower alone. Willpower won't work against a determined ego voice.

Eventually, you cave in and grab whatever handy rationale the ego offers you, and you drink. Relief will flood in, and the discomfort will dissipate as soon as you make the decision, perhaps even before you've taken the action. And it feels great! For a bit. Then it doesn't, and the same thing happens that always happens. You wake up in the stuck place, and you remember what you had conveniently forgotten: you *hate* the stuck place. It's awful, as it's not what you want; this is not where you want to be. Yet here you are. You feel regret and disappointment and are angry at yourself. Then you wake up one morning and feel the calling again. Then the whole cycle repeats itself. Have you done this?

Many of my clients have done this several times, and each time they have felt like a loser or that there is something wrong with them. When we keep failing in this way it just reinforces the limiting beliefs we have about ourselves. *See, you can't do it. You will only fail again. You keep messing up. You are going to fail, so why bother*, the ego voice says.

The ego can kick in at different points for people when they first stop drinking, but it will really ramp up when the ego contemplates that this "sobriety thing" is a "forever thing." And that is too terrifying for the ego to comprehend. A whole life without alcohol? What does that mean? Remember we have invested a lot of energy into what we believe alcohol *means* for us. It is the promise of alcohol, what we think it means in our lives, that makes it feel so distressing to give up. The ego is fully signed up and on board with the messaging that alcohol means something, we need to have it, and it's not fair if we can't. And this is how we self-sabotage our calling.

Here are some steps for preventing ego sabotage:

1. Ask yourself, *What is real here, and what is a story I am making up?*

2. Reassure yourself that this is not an emergency, and you are safe.

3. Journal about why you want to make these changes, so you can stay clear on your intention to change.

4. Make a list of all the times you have felt fear and discomfort but have kept going anyway.

BREAKING THROUGH OUR UPPER LIMITS

In *The Big Leap* Gay Hendricks refers to the resistance we hit as our "upper limits."[6] We all have these, and we have them in every area of our lives. We will always, without fail, hit an upper limit when we grow. And getting sober *is* growth. What no one has told you until now is that resistance, the ego, and upper limits can all be overcome when you know how. It is simply a life skill that we can develop.

We hit upper limits in every area of our lives because we are always growing. We have haphazardly navigated past some of them and have stumbled at others. I have always hit an upper limit whenever I engage in any formal education. It is a well-established pattern with me. I am dyslexic, but it wasn't diagnosed until I was in my first year of college. I always knew I wasn't stupid, but I did stupid things. There are words I would repeatedly not be able to spell, and I would feel ashamed and embarrassed. When I started my degree, or whenever I started a new semester, I would always go through intense fear and panic. My ego would go into overdrive and would say things like, *You can't do this. You're going to fail, and people will realize you are an idiot. You will show yourself up.* And I would feel an intense need to quit and run so no one would discover that I can't spell and have no idea where to put a comma.

Somehow, I would muddle through. Alcohol probably numbed me to the fear and discomfort, and I soldiered on. And then whatever course I was doing would eventually become familiar and would feel a bit easier. Then the ego would begin to relax, the fear would subside, and I would begin to feel that I could do it. I've never failed a course. I didn't always get spectacular grades, but somehow I got through. Somehow, I managed to overcome the upper limit and grow into whatever it was I was learning. When the new thing becomes a familiar thing the ego voice calms down. The same thing will happen with sobriety.

You have probably had similar experiences. We have all developed methods to get through our upper limits. We have muddled through, often sabotaging ourselves unnecessarily. When you understand that resistance and upper limits are just part of the growth process, you can then navigate around them with less effort and stress and achieve better results.

Imagine your upper limit is like a wall. On the other side of it is a new experience, one that will enrich and change you, help you to grow. Some of it may be tough, some of it might be glorious, but growing into this new experience on the other side of your upper limit is what you were designed to do, what you are *called* to do. What often happens, though, is that once we get to a place that feels comfortable, we don't have the same motivation to push through the upper limit. We become complacent and will often talk ourselves out of change (growth) because we don't want to go through the upper limit. So, we stay stuck in the same place, be it a job, relationship, or circumstances that are no longer working for us, simply because change feels too hard.

Our upper limits are very much shaped by our limiting beliefs—the faulty beliefs we created when we were processing information as children. Because as children we didn't have the self-awareness to challenge the belief systems we were creating, we absorbed them without applying any critical thinking. The work of adulthood is to do that critical thinking, so we can grow. We all have limiting beliefs. We all have upper limits policed by the ego voice, and we all experience fear and resistance when we are called to grow. But by doing this work we can develop a sober mindset. Kelly Ruta, a mindset strategist and keynote speaker, taught me the following:

> It is part of every human's experience to bump up against limiting beliefs, upper limits, and the ego constantly trying to keep us in a safe little box. Until you learn the skills to navigate this it is nearly impossible to blow that box to pieces and step into the fullness of your life, your relationships, and your work. The fact that we don't learn the skills early on in life is tragic, but the good news is you can learn them now and support your sobriety and your dreams for the rest of your life.[7]

Here are some steps for getting past your upper limits:

1. Get into your body and notice how you are feeling.

2. Pay attention to the story your ego voice is telling you. Example: *This isn't a good idea, you will fail, everyone will laugh.*

3. Acknowledge to yourself that this is the ego voice just trying to keep you safe; it is not the voice of all-knowing truth.

4. Journal and talk to someone you trust as this helps us get perspective.

5. Let go of the outcome and focus on the next right action.
   Example: *I can't control what will happen here or how this will work out. All I can do is my best and ask for help when I need it.*

6. Take the next right action and then the next one after that and the next one after that.
   Example: *I'll send the email, then I'll write a list, then I'll submit the application.*

7. Repeat this process as often as necessary.

LIMITING BELIEFS

In this section I want to outline how limiting beliefs are formed, why they are important, and why in sobriety we must keep working on uncovering and changing them.

Our limiting beliefs are very common because we are not even remotely original. The thoughts that used to limit me probably limit you too. Although we will have many limiting beliefs, they can often be boiled down to a handful of fundamental ones that govern our lives. Two of my fundamental limiting beliefs were *I'm not good enough* and *I won't be loved.* I believed that these were true, in the same way that I believed the sun would set at night.

Limiting beliefs become rules that reside in our subconscious minds. They are like mantras—they vibrate within us, and we repeat them over and over to ourselves, searching for evidence to reinforce them. These rules shape the experience we have in the world, and most of us have no idea they are even there.

Because our brains are constantly processing information, they need to do this as efficiently as possible. So, our brains create a filter system, a bit like a sieve, really. This allows our brains to sort through the information coming in and process it in a way that means something to us, so we know how to respond.

An example of this would be if you felt left out a lot as a child. Perhaps you didn't get invited to a party or feel included on the playground. Maybe this happened a few times. Because you were a child, you lacked self-awareness and critical thinking, so maybe you began to think, *What's wrong with me? Why doesn't anyone want to play with me?* And a belief system about being included and liked will begin to form.

Fast-forward thirty years, and you're at work. You don't want to drink anymore, but this means saying no to after-work drinks. You know that if you go you will feel tempted to drink, and you don't want that, but you will also feel left out if you don't go. In fact, the more you think about it, the more it seems like *everyone* is having fun at the bar after work, and you are the sad lonely loser no one really likes, who is going home. Your ego voice will be telling you a familiar story about why you are left out. Your filter system will take this information and say, *Friends are having fun without you* and link it to a time in the past when you felt left out when you were younger. This will kick off an emotional reaction that you will feel in your body and that will then kick off subsequent thoughts linked to those emotions. The thinking and feeling will work in tandem, so the ego message feels true. The ego voice will be saying things like, *See, they don't really like you. They put up with you, but no one really cares, and they are not going to miss you. You will always be alone. If you drink, you will have friends, because people who drink are carefree and fun.* The ego judges your *present* experience like a *past* experience because of the faulty beliefs you created in the past that are now hidden in your subconscious mind.

Remember that the ego and subconscious mind are working together to make sense of the current experience as efficiently as possible. *This* is like *that*. And because feeling left out as a kid felt so devastating, the perception of feeling left out as an adult feels equally devastating. We are reexperiencing past pain. These responses are automatic and happen on autopilot. We are already feeling the emotions in our bodies before our rational mind can kick in and say, *Being sober is the most important thing right now. When you feel secure, you can go along for an hour or two. You have lots of friends who like doing things with you that don't involve alcohol.*

We all have our own version of this type of scenario playing out in our minds. Think back to when you had an irrational or unbalanced response to a seemingly minor or inconsequential event. Our filter systems will identify current experiences and link them to past ones. We then start telling ourselves a familiar story about ourselves, one that usually makes us feel bad and reinforces our negative feelings.

The thing about this story is that it feels very real—it feels like it's a fact. When we have the awareness of what is happening, we can begin to change the story and challenge the ego voice and limiting beliefs. We can observe our feelings and thoughts and notice our response. We can interrupt this cycle by asking simple questions like, *Is this true?* Employ your rational mind and say, *Well, it's not totally true. I do have friends who want to do stuff that's not based on alcohol, and I've heard a few colleagues complain about their hangovers and look embarrassed when the previous night's activities have been discussed. So maybe they are not having as much fun as I think they are. I know I don't want to feel like that again.*

We want our rational mind to challenge the automatic story our subconscious mind is telling us about the event. When we do this, we will shift our mindset to something more helpful and progressive. This is why this work is so essential. Working on our mindset is not exclusive to people with an alcohol problem—it is essential to *all* human beings. It's just that most people don't realize it. It is pain that motivates us to change. It's only when our relationship with alcohol becomes uncomfortable enough that we look to change it. And this is the good news.

This program is not about just getting rid of the pain, it's about personal development work that leads to a glorious expansive life. That's the bonus we get. It doesn't matter how much you are drinking or how little, by quitting you get the space and energy to grow. That's why my friend Laura McKowen coined the hashtag #wearetheluckiest. How lucky are we that alcohol has pushed us to a place where we can do this deeper, life-changing work? Without my alcohol problem I may have lived my whole life just existing in the external world, never knowing who I am and what I am capable of. I could have missed my own life.

The stories we tell ourselves are painful, but they are not who we are. The greatest tragedy is how we can spend our whole lives believing what the ego tells us about ourselves. Uncovering and changing our limiting beliefs is one of the most liberating and empowering experiences we can have. It is also essential to your sobriety and your ability to get sober in the first place.

Here are some steps to uncovering your limiting beliefs:

1. The best way to discover your limiting beliefs is to pay attention to your critical voice. How do you speak about yourself? What are the phrases you use over and over?
   Example: *I'm so stupid. I'll never be able to finish that. I'm only going to mess it up so why bother trying.*

2. Journal about where these beliefs came from. Did someone speak to you in this way? How did your parents criticize you?

   Example: *I was always told I was messy or that I couldn't do things.*

3. Now that you have identified your limiting beliefs, change them into something that is more honest and empowering.

   Example: *It's okay to mess up. I learn a lot about myself when I do. I am open to learning new things. I'm going to go step-by-step and ask for help when I need it.*

4. Notice how these new beliefs feel better. They are closer to the truth than the limiting ones.

5. Repeat new beliefs every time a limiting belief gets triggered.

CHANGING OUR STORY

Because we live so much of our day on autopilot, with this chatter in our heads, the first step to changing it is to bring our awareness to it. Observe what the ego is saying. It's usually a pretty consistent message. Self-awareness is one of the greatest tools we have to push back against the ego. When difficult or uncomfortable feelings kick in, ask, *Is this true? How do I know this is true? Where did this belief about myself come from?* When you do this, you are starting the process of dismantling the story that has kept you limited.

We confuse truth with perception. How we perceive things is not always as they are. Let's say, for example, you were the child on the playground who was feeling left out. The kids are playing a game they really enjoy. A couple of them waved for you to come over, but you felt too shy. The kids in the game interpreted that to mean you weren't interested and carried on with what they were doing. It wasn't personal. If they had been older or had better communication skills, maybe they could have been more persistent. But all that happened in this event was a small miscommunication. How it was perceived, however, was entirely different. And this is how our filter system begins to be created.

With some examination, we can find that things we thought were true, like *I'm not good enough*, are actually our perception of events. Because our brain is sorting through data as quickly as possible, we repeatedly think *this is like that*, when actually it is nothing of the sort. When we employ our self-awareness, the opposite of being on autopilot, we can begin to question and reflect on what is true for us and what isn't. We want to shake the foundations of these limiting beliefs that we have formed. They will crumble because they are not based on any truth.

Journal Prompts to Start Uncovering and Understanding Your Own Limiting Beliefs in Relation to Sobriety.

When you think of what sobriety means, what does the voice (the ego) in your head say?

> Example: *Sobriety is boring. Sobriety is hard. You won't have fun again. You won't have any friends if you don't drink.*

Are these things true? Where do they come from?

> Example: *I have no idea where these beliefs come from; I've just always had them and thought they were facts. But considering all the sober people I have seen online, maybe it's possible that sobriety is different from how I imagine it is.*

What does that voice in your head say when you do something new?

Example: *I am going to fail. I can't do this. I will make mistakes, so I shouldn't even bother.*

Is it possible that some of the things you believe about yourself may not actually be true? How does that make you feel?

Example: *Yes, it's possible. I can see how my thinking defeats me.*

...

THE MAIN EVENT

Growth is messy, and it can be frustrating, but it is always worth it. The most significant action you can take to aid your own growth is to get out of your own damn way. That is why in this chapter we took a deep dive into the ways you sabotage your own growth.

In the chapter on movement, we discussed being purposeful about the direction of our lives, and that is very linked to the idea of growth. When we move toward something purposeful, we want it to be authentic and meaningful. Authenticity is essential to growth. The ego voice is not our authentic self, so if we listen to it we are in danger of putting lots of energy into moving toward something that isn't aligned with who we really are.

It's very easy to get lost in the details of life and miss the main event. Drinking alcohol is a very insignificant detail, and yet for some of us it becomes the main event, and we lose ourselves. However much bandwidth we are sacrificing to alcohol is too much. We don't have to drink because other people expect it, and we don't have to drink so much that it takes over our lives.

Our main event is to grow, and the world needs you to grow into the person you are capable of being.

When I say that growth never stops, what I mean is that the things I struggled with twenty years ago, ten years ago, or even one year ago are not the same things I struggle with now. For years I lived my life believing I wasn't good enough. I made all my decisions based on this limiting belief. When I did the process work to uncover it, understand it, and get free of it, I saw everything differently. I got different outcomes. Struggling with a feeling of not being good enough is not my challenge today. I have other challenges because I am growing. This is just how the human experience works. What is different is I have the understanding and knowledge to manage the challenges.

These new mindset skills are vital to our growth and purpose—our main event. Getting drunk, being hungover, and thinking about or planning to drink are not—I repeat, *are not*—part of your main event.

DON'T MISS YOUR LIFE

No one knows how to get from point A to point Z. Not even the supersmart people who are successful. Point A is the starting point. Square one. Some of us may know how to get from A to E or sometimes just from A to B. It doesn't really matter. What does matter is that you start where you are. Everything we do leads to something else. It's cause and effect. Getting sober will lead to something else—something better. Use the bandwidth you have in sobriety to listen to your calling. Trust me that this is a trial-and-error process. The mistakes you make are glorious growth opportunities. The life I have now is a result of all my failures. The ego voice will take failure and try to make it something bad—it will present it as a reason for not trying and for not changing.

Remember there is no such thing as failure—only feedback. Focus on the feedback, especially if it's uncomfortable, because within it is the tool you need to get to the next square. Having a vision and a goal is great, but we also have to keep focusing on moving toward the next square. Each square we travel to will probably throw up some resistance—so the more practice we have in navigating the ego voice and getting over our upper limits, the better.

Through practice, we will get better and better at identifying the difference between our calling and the ego voice. What I want for you more than anything is for you not to miss your life and not to waste the time and energy managing alcohol. What saddens me the most about the rampant alcohol abuse that is tearing through our culture is the loss of potential. The could-have-beens, but weren't. Listen to your calling no matter how uncomfortable that is and lean into the growth. Because your growth is the main event.

What really matters to you?

> Example: *My family. Time with people I care about and who nourish me. My work.*

If you got all this bandwidth back because you were sober, what would you do with it?

> Example: *I would spend less time worrying about things I've done. I'd have more time to study, work, be with my kids, and exercise.*

What is your main event?

> Example: *Serving others, being creative, being a great parent, building my business, getting my degree, being open to opportunities.*

...

Conclusion

The five pillars do not exist in isolation; rather, they are interconnected. If one isn't connected or doesn't work, the others won't either. The synchronicity will break down. Personal development is not something we do once and then are done with. Managing our mental, emotional, and spiritual health is a lifelong process.

The five pillars are really personal development for us all, sober or otherwise. Everyone on the planet would benefit from personal development—the development of one's character—but not everyone knows this. You may have felt that the idea of not drinking again is the worst thing that has ever happened to you. But it may just be that quitting drinking is going to push you into personal development work that you would never have done otherwise. Ironically, your drinking could give you a life-changing opportunity. Grab it. This work will transform your life in ways you didn't imagine possible. We don't do this work to stay away from a drink one day at a time. We do it so we can live enriched, purposeful, amazing lives free from the need for alcohol. The five pillars are how we get across the bridge from the land of alcohol to the land of sobriety.

As you may have noticed as you read this book, the focus was not on tips and tricks to stay away from alcohol. Breaking the habit of drinking alcohol is the first requirement, and that can

feel tough at the beginning. But our efforts can't end there—
that would be denying ourselves the best part of this whole deal.
Sobriety is about gaining freedom in our minds, stability in our
emotions, and the bandwidth to expand into a life we want to
live, not one we want to escape from. Working this program is
how you can achieve that. Remember, the problem is within us,
but so is the solution.

WE BEHAVE HOW WE FEEL

Human behavior is a window into our inner life. An easy way to
tell what is going on inside someone is to look at what they *do*.
Our feelings will, to a large extent, dictate our actions. And our
actions will always have consequences. After all, life is a study
of consequences. All of us come to a point in our lives when we
have the opportunity to ask ourselves, *Why is this happening?*
Why do I feel this way? It's in this moment (often referred to as
a moment of clarity) that we realize we don't want these consequences anymore—that we don't like how we behave. By asking
ourselves these questions, we can find a different path. Changing
our behavior will help a little bit, but because all our behavior
has emotional roots, we have to get to the heart of the problem
to truly transform ourselves.

I have always seen an alcohol problem as a manifestation of much
deeper emotional issues. Alcohol becomes a problem because of
all the stuff underneath it—the unresolved childhood hurts, the
painful relationships, the struggle to find balance, the seemingly
unmanageable feelings and emotions, and the programming in our
subconscious mind. An alcohol abuse problem does not grow out
of nothing. Alcohol has provided our culture with such a quick, effective, socially condoned, and cheap method of damping down
feelings we don't like. Why change when you can just hide behind
alcohol and numb your feelings quickly and cheaply?

Alcohol has promised us solutions to all sorts of problems and a vehicle to a land we all want to go. Who doesn't want to live in The Land and have all the fun, excitement, belonging, connection, relaxation, rewards, and romance? I know I did; I just didn't know how to get there without alcohol. We live in a culture where everything is focused on the "outer," not the "inner." We get lost in the external world and lose who we really are inside.

Alcohol lied to so many of us. It told us that it was a quick outside fix for whatever pain we were feeling and could quickly manufacture the nice feelings. If you are not getting a good return on your investment with alcohol, it's up to you to decide whether to keep plugging away, hoping that one day you'll get the buzz without the consequences. Or, you could quit and try this program. Maybe you could try this sober journey for a year or so. If your life hasn't improved markedly at the end of it, then alcohol is always going to be there. It's never going to go away. But if you do decide to stop, you need to do the personal development work to effect the change and transformation that is possible in sobriety. I often use the phrase "Sobriety is my superpower," and it's really true. Being sober will give you an edge like nothing else. My hope is that after reading this book you know there is a bridge to the land of sobriety. I invite you to cross it now.

THE FIRST THREE PILLARS

When you are getting started in sobriety, focus on the first three pillars. If this is your day one, or you are working toward stopping, just focus on movement. Prioritize exercise in your life. Move your body because you are worth it. Dance around your living room, park your car at the back of the parking lot and walk to where you are going. Any kind of movement will help you feel better. Then ask yourself, *What do I want to move toward?* Listen for your answer. Ask the question over and over. It may feel a little uncomfortable at first if you have been disconnected from yourself and have learned to ignore that voice deep inside you. The feeling of discomfort will ease when you connect to the answer.

Then start thinking about who you have around you. Do you have supportive people around you, or do you have people who will question and push back on your decision to stop drinking? Are your connection needs being met? The first step to meeting these needs is to be aware they exist. We can't solve a problem until we know what the problem is. Where can you find support? What is there locally? You don't have to commit to anything right now—just educate yourself on what support is accessible to you. This may be a time when you opt to spend more time with people who are supportive of you and less with the ones who want every social gathering to involve alcohol. Stopping drinking is a really good way to find out who your friends are. Your real friends will be supportive—your drinking buddies will needle you to start drinking again.

When you stop drinking, everything is going to feel a little out of balance. You live in an alcohol saturated world, so it will feel weird at first. What do you do on a Saturday night when you don't drink? What do you do on a Sunday morning when you are not hungover? How do you socialize without alcohol? Navigating the world without alcohol will seem strange in the beginning, which is why having support is crucial—whether it is support from friends or family, a professional, or a support group. Please don't do this alone. Begin to practice balance and be kind to yourself. Learning how to balance your needs when you've only just become aware that you have needs is a trial-and-error process.

Balance takes practice. The first step is just bringing your awareness to the elements of HALT as discussed. Focus on these four areas of need and practice responding in a way that is healthy. Don't stay up late watching TV if you are tired. Instead, go to bed earlier. Feed your body nutritious food. Call a supportive friend. Listen to your body when you feel anger rising. Ask yourself, *What's really going on here?* You won't get it right all the time, and that is perfectly okay, no one does. It is a practice we are developing.

You will have to think about sobriety. You will have to think about your daily life and how you structure it. You will have to be conscious about your choices. And this will require some energy. A lifestyle shift of this kind is going to require effort because it is unfamiliar, that's all. With time it will become your new normal. Give yourself that time. Perspective is everything. Sobriety can *feel* hard at the beginning, but then it becomes easier. Do you remember those old TV sets where you had to turn the dial to get a station? Sobriety is a bit like that. At first you will see a fuzzy screen, and you just have to keep turning and turning. Some days you will get a picture and others, not so much. But if you keep going no matter what, the picture becomes easier to tune in and gets clearer and clearer. Until one day you realize that the picture is in high-definition color. That's what early sobriety feels like. Just keep tuning in.

THE LAST TWO PILLARS

Process and growth are something you can bring your awareness to when you feel stable in your sobriety. When you get sober, you will receive the call to grow. You can't help but grow, but how you grow will depend on the skills you need to develop in order to navigate the ego and your limiting beliefs and get through your upper limits. The call to growth can be frightening sometimes, as it can often mean change and change in itself is scary for some of us. If we don't drink, everything else in our lives is negotiable—we can change things that don't serve us, let go of the past, and craft a different future. One of the ways we can start to support our growth is through knowledge. We will have the bandwidth to absorb a lot of what we are learning and be able to apply it. Check out the reference section at the back of this book and dive into some of the books I've listed. There are also lots of amazing podcasts out there. You can check out the *Soberful* podcast, of course, but there are lots of other great sober and personal development podcasts too. Breathe in the knowledge. It will aid and equip you in your growth.

But remember that the personal development work of sobriety is not a passive exercise. We can't make ourselves better just by reading or listening. I often have people come to me who have read all the quit lit, listened to all the podcasts, and think that is doing "the work." It's not. It's information and identification. Although that is important, it won't facilitate the internal transformation you are searching for. Remember, if you feel differently you will behave differently. This is why at some point I feel you would benefit from some therapy, coaching, group work, or a self-help program or workshop that helps you dive deeper into your own personal material. Through this you will have light-bulb moments, where you gain insight into yourself, which will lead you to the next square on the board. You will grow in ways you can't imagine right now. Being sober *is* growth—it is a new land with new possibilities. The minute you put down the drink and make a decision to commit to sobriety, you are growing—it is inevitable. Being sober will help you think more clearly and give you the energy to grow into what you are capable of being.

The true essence of growth is "revealing ourselves to ourselves." We can start that with some kind of journaling, either structured or unstructured, as a way to explore our innermost thoughts and feelings. Journaling is a way to have a conversation and therefore a connection with oneself. That's why I included all of the journaling prompts throughout the book. Writing things down focuses us. It also allows us to look back at different times and see our progress. Most importantly, it takes "things" from our heads and gives us a chance to look at them. Remember, it's in our heads that the trouble exists. Writing gets it out. As part of your new sobriety I encourage you to start daily journaling as a way to connect with your inner world.

Process work will also happen very early on, too. When we come out of the fog of the drinking culture we have lived in, we begin to see things differently. We may notice things about ourselves that we didn't before, or we may see ourselves reflected in others and begin to process how and why we behaved the way we did.

Process work is how we understand ourselves and why we are the way we are. Because we have more bandwidth to process stuff when we stop drinking, process work starts when drinking stops. However, be aware that there may be many issues you need to process that require expert support and help. Pace yourself. It's okay to put some issues on the shelf for later when you feel safer and more stable.

Safety is a crucial component to process work. Before we delve into our past, we need to feel a degree of safety in our situation, and with the person we are working with. Be aware of what makes you feel safe and take responsibility for what you need in order to feel safe. It will unfold in its own time and come to you naturally.

Build a foundation for sobriety that is balanced with lots of support, as this will help you when you begin to uncover stuff from your past that may be painful. I used to have a tendency to run away (far, far away) from anything that was painful or uncomfortable. I did not understand why anyone would volunteer to do what I call "emotional heart surgery," or facing your past and your issues head-on. Then it came to my attention just how hard and uncomfortable running away was, not to mention exhausting. Surely there had to be an easier way.

It was then that I realized there was no way to avoid dealing with the pain that I was carrying inside me—the only way through it was *through* it. And that is how we get free. We honor and validate the pain we carry within. We take the lessons from it so our past can be transformed into wisdom. And when we are free, we won't want to numb or run anymore.

OUR LIFE'S WORK

The work of emotional sobriety lasts our lifetime. We are our life's work. We get ourselves right first, then we can be of use/help to others by just being ourselves. At the time of this writing, I am over twenty years sober. I don't do this work so that I don't drink. I simply never think about drinking or not drinking. I do this work because of the rewards it brings. The personal development work I have been describing has not only enabled my life to expand—it has helped me deal with the challenges I've faced. I am someone who has always wanted more. It's just that the stuff I want more of now is (mostly) good stuff.

Sobriety will help you become a better version of yourself. We are all "becoming," and we never really stop. It's an ongoing process. There is no destination, only the journey, because there is always more to *be*. Each stage of life is an opportunity to become more if we allow it. Allowing is the optimal word here, as we are all capable of getting in our own way.

This book was never about trying to persuade you to stop drinking; it was about facilitating your awakening to what is possible if you change your relationship with alcohol and introduce simple practices to make sobriety sustainable for you.

ALCOHOL: A PREDETERMINED RELATIONSHIP

Our relationship with alcohol is complicated, messy, often abusive, and hard to untangle from. What is astounding to me is that it's always *presumed* we will have a relationship with alcohol. It's just what grown-ups do. I think in Western culture we are conditioned to think this way from a young age. There is an inevitability to alcohol use. In particular, binge drinking is presented as the best way to have fun, and the consequences of binge drinking are deliberately obscured—to our detriment. Therefore, it is the dishonest representation of alcohol use as harmless that I object to the most, not the actual drinking itself.

Was being alcohol-free ever presented to you as a lifestyle option? Unless our religion requires us to abstain, we are raised to expect that we will drink alcohol one day. We may not be directly told this, but it is modeled all around us. It's almost like we had no choice. We didn't actually choose to drink—we just assumed that's what everyone does, so we did: "There are lots of things that are going to happen when you are an adult. You will get a driver's license and a job and earn your own money and, oh, drink alcohol. That's just how it is."

What I would like is for alcohol use and its consequences to be represented much more honestly. What I want the narrative to be is this: Some people choose to drink alcohol. In moderation this can be pleasurable; however, even the smallest amount of alcohol consumption will have consequences, so you need to decide if the cost is worth the benefit. It is not necessary to drink alcohol in order to have fun and feel like you belong.

I would like not drinking to be a legitimate choice just like vegetarianism. Forty years ago, if you were vegetarian or vegan, you were looked at strangely. It was a fringe hippie thing. You might be lucky and get an omelet or a salad, but no one really catered to you. Now, I can be gluten-free, dairy-free, nut-free, and vegan, and no one bats an eye. Your dietary restrictions and requirements will be accommodated. Your choice is respected and understood. But alcohol-free? People will still look at you sideways.

Being alcohol-free or not drinking is different from being sober. People who are alcohol-free or just don't drink have made a lifestyle choice as they can see the benefits. Being sober is different; it means no longer being drunk, no longer self-sabotaging, no more self-destructing. Sober is about *before* and *after*. It's about seeing a choice, a lifestyle that is attractive, and purposefully claiming it. I would like alcohol-free to be as accepted and understood and normalized as being vegetarian is. I would like not drinking to be presented as a lifestyle option, and I would like sobriety to be something that is open and celebrated.

I got to know the creator of a movie called *A Royal Hangover* a few years ago.[1] It was directed by a young man named Arthur Cauty, who was only about twenty-seven at the time. He was a professional filmmaker who was interested in the British relationship with binge drinking. He didn't drink, although he had two older brothers who did. Choosing not to drink alcohol is greeted with deep suspicion in the UK, as I know it is in many Western cultures. That's especially true when you are in your teens and twenties. I asked him what it was like when he was at school and how his peer group responded to his not drinking. He shrugged and said, "I was just the weird one."[2]

He explained that as a teenager, he was busy with martial arts and exploring filmmaking. He didn't have time to drink and saw his older brothers wrecked and hungover and thought it was incredibly unattractive, so he just didn't drink. I admired his self-esteem and courage to go against the tide, as it couldn't have been easy. It made me sad that he was called weird because he didn't want to get drunk on alcohol. It also made me think about all of the other young people who may not have had the self-esteem or courage to resist the peer and cultural pressure. Often people find that it's easier to just join in rather than feel left out.

Needing to belong is such a powerful motivator when we are young. My mission is to create a world where "not drinking alcohol" is like being gluten-free. It's a choice people make for various reasons, including health, but mostly because they want full access to their bandwidth and what life has to offer. If you are gluten-free, no one starts pressuring you to eat bread. People don't say, "Here, have a breadstick—just one won't hurt." But if you are alcohol-free, people don't understand, and they challenge your choice. Nondrinkers have to justify themselves, as alcohol users simply can't understand why anyone would willingly decide not to drink if they didn't have a problem.

Being sober is more understood. People think that if you have a problem you have to stop, poor you. But not drinking as a lifestyle choice is baffling to the wider culture. We have to change this. We have to change our culture. What I am asking for is a more honest conversation about our relationship with alcohol and its cultural representations. I want our culture to honestly portray the costs of drinking alcohol and not just the perceived benefits. I want to see representations of an alcohol-free lifestyle, so we can show that no one is missing out on anything just because they don't drink.

We need to create a different narrative around alcohol, one that serves people rather than deceives them. On average, people try for ten years to manage their relationship with alcohol before giving up and getting sober[3]—a whole decade with alcohol as their main event. And the main reason for this, as I have discussed throughout this book, is the misguided belief that they will have to give up going to The Land if they stop. Sobriety is not joyless, as we are led to believe, it's an amazing revelation.

This is why so many people are becoming more and more public about their sobriety. On blogs, podcasts, and Instagram accounts, there are more and more people saying, "I'm sober and who knew it could be this friggin' good!" More and more people are awakening to the fact that a sober, alcohol-free life can bring you so much more than you ever imagined.

I hope this book has given you a pathway to the life that you deserve. I hope you get some help, try the five pillars, and give sobriety a chance. Remember that nothing has to be done perfectly. Good enough will get you where you need to go. Please don't think you are struggling alone. You are not. What I have been telling you throughout this book is the great big sober secret: you can get to The Land of fun, excitement, belonging, connection, relaxation, rewards, and romance without alcohol. And guess what? It's better. All of those things are better sober. That's the secret. Many of us have crossed the bridge and live joyously in the land of sobriety. There are all sorts of communities now with a place for you. Claim it and claim the life that is waiting for you.

ACKNOWLEDGMENTS

This book has been twenty years in the making, and it all really started with Chip Somers, who gave me my first job as a therapist. I can now see how lucky I was to learn and train with him and the incredible team at Focus12. Chip has been my boss, mentor, and friend and is currently my podcast cohost. Thank you for continuing to take chances on me.

I love the name "Soberful" and all it represents, but I can't take credit for dreaming it up. It was Mindee Clem Forman who did, and I will be forever grateful.

Annemarie Young—I can't write without you; you make my words so much better. I am in deep gratitude of your friendship and professionalism, and I promise not to swear in books anymore.

Tony Robinson—My man in Cambridge. Do as she says.

Diane Simone—Thank you from the bottom of my heart for helping me sort out my references. You have no idea how much time, trouble, and frustration you saved me. This book would never have been submitted without your help.

Tasha Kelter—Thank you for your outstanding services in editing. You are so helpful to this dyslexic writer.

My agent, Stephanie Tade—You had me at hello. I had total faith that the perfect agent would appear and would get what I was trying to do with this book. And you did. Thank you for your belief in this project.

My editor, Diana Ventimiglia—I can't thank you enough for believing and championing this book and pushing me to make it better. I promise to do all I can to make it as great as I can.

Sounds True is just the perfect publisher for my book, and I am so honored to be in your world. Thank you for your attention to detail and the fine-tuning and excellent editing of this book.

Will Weisser—Thank you for helping me pull together such a great book proposal and introducing me to such a fabulous agent.

Laura Wright—Thank God I found you. You made me dream big and see what was possible for the Soberful program. I love how you are leading women to smash through their limits and create heart-centered businesses that serve others. Raise your banners, and I will attend as I am in your debt.

Kelly Ruta, queen of badassery—Thank you for being a qualified leader in the field of mindset. I have learned so much from you, and it has informed so much of my work in addiction. I wait with anticipation for your mindset book!

Craig Weiner and Alina Frank—Thank you for being pioneers of EFT and providing a safe and solid place to train and grow.

The Soberful team who support me and champion this work. You make it possible for me to go out and do my thing.

Louise O'Brien—My God, how did I do it before you came and saved me? You are the best assistant a woman could have. How have we not met in person? I feel like you are my family. Please don't leave me ever.

Tamara Kirby—You are amazing to me, from where you were to where you are now. I am in awe and value our friendship deeply.

Mimi Divine Touhey—Your skills are a great addition to the team, and I think your work around women's hormones and sobriety is really important.

Yulonda Ross—Thank you for being a great team member; I could listen to your accent all day.

Jan Bowen and Leeny Barrett—Thank you so much for being such wonderful supporters on the Facebook group and such great advocates for the Soberful program.

All our wonderful Facebook moderators (you know who you are)—I love seeing you grow.

Jamey Jones—Thank you for writing fantastic copy and really getting me. You are a pleasure to work with.

Britany Felix—Thank you for helping me make the podcast the success it has become.

Paul and Alexandra Stennett—Thank you for doing such an excellent job with the editing and promotion of the podcast.

Danielle Fitzpatrick Clark—Thank you for your beautiful work and helping me grow this thing.

Fiona Smallwood—Thank you for all your efforts in getting the message across. I have loved seeing your awakening.

Sylvie Longstreet and Carolyne Etherington—Thanks for doing all the things that I am terrible at, brilliantly.

Lou, Jan, Leeny, Collen, Libby, and Joe—Thank you for reading the manuscript and giving me some honest, detailed feedback. It was helpful beyond anything you could imagine.

Grachelle Sherburne—Thank you for your guidance and support in ensuring that the Soberful program is inclusive and welcoming to all.

Melissa Anne—Thank you so much for your help and support. I never would have finished this book if you weren't there looking after my kids during the pandemic.

Linzi Treby and Emma Gawlinski—My lifelong friends and sisters.

Florence Miller—I will always treasure our friendship; you mean the world to me.

Sarah Gillespie—My soul sister. I can't imagine traversing this life without your observations and insights. Thank you for allowing us to use your beautiful music as our podcast intro. It was perfect, and you are the most talented and compassionate woman I know.

Theresa Hardy—You probably have no idea what a lifeline you were for me when I nursed my two babies. You made me feel safe and cared for. Thank you for that and for championing how important it is to nurse your baby.

Beth Yendrick—You were my first real mum friend. I'm so glad our boys liked each other just as much as we did/do.

Oyster Bay Power Girls Mimi Bishop, Amy Basnight, and Carly Clark Zimmer—You were a lifeline when I was so lonely; I'm holding you all to the spa retreat in the Hamptons!

Jeane LaRance—Your kindness helped me so much in the early days. I love you and miss you. Rest in peace.

Karen Luknis and Mary Gauthier—You two were very inspiring to me in my first months of sobriety. Thank you for creating a safe environment for me when I first got sober.

Joe Schrank—You drive me crazy and are the best at what you do.

John and Sue Jones—This book is full of your wisdom; thank you for your ongoing love and support. You are my family.

The online sober world: Khadi Olagoke, Kristi Coulter, Laurie Dhue, Anna David, Kelly Fitzgerald, Annie Grace, Mandy Manners and Kate Baily, Lucy Rocca, Laura Willoughby, Lotta Dan, Africa Brook, Joanne Bradford, Lara Frazier, Laura Silverman, Julie Maida, Jennifer Matisse, Laura McKowen, Holly Whitikar, and so many more—Thank you for everything you bring. For too long sobriety had to be a secret, shameful thing. Seeing so many women emerge with blogs, podcasts, and Instagram accounts to tell their stories has been incredible to witness. Let's continue to show the world what a great thing sobriety can be. There are different paths that all lead to the same place, and we need all of them as there are still so many people who have no idea how incredible this life can be. We are changing the world.

Dawn and Taryn of SHE RECOVERS—Special thanks to you. You did an amazing thing for so many women—your events are so fun and necessary. I'm happy to be in your tribe.

Adrienne Miller and the Women for Sobriety crew—I love you ladies. Keep growing!

Lynn Matti—Colleague, friend, dancing partner, and zombie apocalypse companion (we have a plan).

Sherry Gaba—You do incredible work helping the affected others. Thank you for your friendship.

Olivia Pennelle—You make being British in America so much fun and are a wonderful asset to the sober community.

Soberful Life members—Thank you. You are truly an inspiration to me. I love seeing you put effort into this sober thing and grow into all you can be. Being with you in our group is my favorite thing to do.

My mum—The older I get, the more I can see of you in me. I love you, and thank you for being a wonderful grandmother.

My family in England—I have learned so many valuable lessons from you.

Mountain Mamas—I am so proud to be your family. You are inspiring and majestic, and I'm happy we are finally in the same time zone.

My stepdaughter, Amanda, and son-in-law, Dustin—It's so great to live so close by. Thank you for making me a grandparent! I am glad my kids will know their older siblings and now their nephew, Jamie.

My stepson, Matthew, and his girlfriend, Lauren—It is such a joy to be part of this beautiful blended family. Thank you for being so great with the boys and always calling me on my birthday.

Cadbury—I never knew I was a dog lover until I met you!

My husband, Rob—I can only be all of this because of you. It's your belief and love for me that is my greatest strength. Thank you for taking the boys on all the days I've had to hide out in hotels, so I have the space to write and think.

My darling ones, Xavier and Lukey—Being your mummy is the best job in the whole wide world. Thank you for choosing me. I will always love you more.

RESOURCES

Here is a comprehensive list of resources with websites to explore.

IN-PERSON AND ONLINE GROUPS

Alcoholics Anonymous (aa.org)—Self-help spiritual program

Celebrate Recovery (celebraterecovery.com)—Christian-based recovery

Jewish Alcoholics, Chemically Dependent Persons, and Significant Others (JACS) (jewishboard.org)

Life Recovery (liferecoverygroups.com)—Faith-based recovery

LifeRing (lifering.org)—Secular recovery

Millati Islami (millatiislami.org)—Islamic-based twelve-step recovery

Recovery Dharma (recoverydharma.org)—Buddhism-based recovery

Refuge Recovery (refugerecovery.org)—Buddhism-based recovery

SHE RECOVERS (sherecovers.org)—Online and in-person support groups for women

SMART Recovery (smartrecovery.org)—Mutual support program

The Phoenix (thephoenix.org)—Gyms for sober people

Transforming Youth Recovery (transformingyouthrecovery.org)—Prevention, education, and support for young people

Wellbriety Movement (wellbriety.com)—A sustainable grassroots movement that provides culturally based healing for the next seven generations of Indigenous people

Women for Sobriety (womenforsobriety.org)—Sobriety program for women

ONLINE SUPPORT

Club Soda (joinclubsoda.com)—UK-based; online with in-person meetups

Gay & Sober (gayandsober.org)—Online resources for the LGBTQ community

Hello Sunday Morning (hellosundaymorning.org)—Australia-based online resource

Sansbar (thesansbar.com)—Traveling pop-up alcohol-free bar experience

Sober Black Girls Club (soberblackgirlsclub.com)—Online and in-person support groups for women of color

Soberful Life (soberful.com/soberful-life/)—Global online subscription group led by addiction professionals

Soberistas (soberistas.com)—UK-based; online with in-person meetups

The Tempest (jointempest.com)—Online support group

EMOTIONAL FREEDOM TECHNIQUE RESOURCES

EFT International (eftinternational.org)

EFT Tapping Training Institute (efttappingtraining.com)

The Tapping Solution (thetappingsolution.com)

RELATIONSHIP RESOURCES

Codependent No More by Melody Beattie

Facing Love Addiction by Pia Mellody

Sex in Recovery by Jennifer Matesa

NOTES

Chapter 1: How Do I Know If I Should Stop or Not?

1. Holly Whitaker, *Quit Like a Woman: The Radical Choice to Not Drink in a Culture Obsessed with Alcohol* (London: Bloomsbury, 2021).
2. Jemma Lennox et al., "The Role of Alcohol in Constructing Gender and Class Identities among Young Women in the Age of Social Media," *The International Journal of Drug Policy* 58 (2018): 13–21, doi.org/10.1016.j.drugpo.2018.04.009.
3. Grachelle Sherburne, personal communication, 2020.
4. Jill Lynne Russett, "Women's Perceptions of High Risk Drinking: Understanding Binge Drinking in a Gender Biased Setting," W&M ScholarWorks (website), 2008, dx.doi.org/doi: 10.25774/w4-aygt-cb32.
5. Derek Kenji Iwamoto et al., "'Man-Ing' up and Getting Drunk: The Role of Masculine Norms, Alcohol Intoxication and Alcohol-Related Problems among College Men," *Addictive Behaviors* 36, no. 9 (September, 2011), doi.org/10.1016/j.addbeh.2011.04.005.

Chapter 4: The Five Pillars of Sustainable Sobriety

1. Benjamin Hardy, *Willpower Doesn't Work: Discover the Hidden Keys to Success.* (Hachette Book Group, 2019).
2. Marcelo R. Roxo et al., "The Limbic System Conception and Its Historical Evolution," *The Scientific World Journal* 11, no. 11 (2011): 2427–40, doi.org/10.1100/2011/157150.
3. Rachael Jack, Oliver G. B. Garrod, and Philippe G. Schyns, "Dynamic Facial Expressions of Emotion Transmit an Evolving Hierarchy of Signals over Time," *Current Biology* 24, no. 2 (January 20, 2014): 187–92, doi.org/10.1016/j.cub.2013.11.064.
4. Dean Mobbs et al., "The Ecology of Human Fear: Survival Optimization and the Nervous System," *Frontiers in Neuroscience*, March 18, 2015, doi.org/10.3389/fnins.2015.00055.

5. Antonio R. Damasio, "Feeling Our Emotions," interview by Manuela Lenzen, *Scientific American*, April 1, 2005, scientificamerican.com/article/feeling-our-emotions/.

6. Peter Clapp, Sanjiv V. Bhave, and Paula L. Hoffman, "How Adaptation of the Brain to Alcohol Leads to Dependence: A Pharmacological Perspective," *Alcohol Research & Health: The Journal of the National Institute on Alcohol Abuse and Alcoholism* 31, no. 4 (2008): 310–39, pubmed.ncbi.nlm.nih.gov/20729980.

7. Steven E. Hyman, Robert C. Malenka, and Eric J. Nestler, "Neural Mechanisms of Addiction: The Role of Reward-Related Learning and Memory," *Annual Review of Neuroscience* 29, no. 1 (July 21, 2006): 565–98, doi.org/10.1146/annurev.neuro.29 .051605.113009.

Chapter 5: The Pillar of Movement

1. Kelly McGonigal, *The Joy of Movement: How Exercise Helps Us Find Happiness, Hope, Connection, and Courage* (New York: Avery, 2019).

2. Tzu-Wei Lin and Yu-Min Kuo, "Exercise Benefits Brain Function: The Monoamine Connection," *Brain Sciences* 3, no. 1 (January 11, 2013): 39–53, doi:10.3390/brainsci3010039.

3. Judith Grisel, *Never Enough: The Neuroscience and Experience of Addiction* (New York: Anchor Books, 2020), 93.

4. Grisel, *Never Enough*, 95.

5. Sukhes Mukherjee, "Alcoholism and Its Effects on the Central Nervous System," *Current Neurovascular Research* 10, no. 3 (2013): 256–62, doi.org/10.2174/15672026113109990004.

6. Joseph M. Boden and David M. Fergusson, "Alcohol and Depression," *Addiction* 106, no. 5 (March 7, 2011): 906–14, doi.org/10.1111/j.1360-0443.2010.03351.x.

7. McGonigal, *The Joy of Movement*, 56.

8. McGonigal, *The Joy of Movement*, 57.

9. Marilyn Freimuth, Sandy Moniz, and Shari R. Kim, "Clarifying Exercise Addiction: Differential Diagnosis, Co-Occurring Disorders, and Phases of Addiction," *International Journal of Environmental Research and Public Health* 8, no. 10 (October 8, 2011): 4070, doi.org/10.3390/ijerph8104069.

10. Barb Carr, "Live Your Core Values: 10-Minute Exercise to Increase Your Success," TapRoot, April 11, 2013, taproot.com /live-your-core-values-exercise-to-increase-your-success/.

Chapter 6: The Pillar of Connection

1. Laura Markham, *Peaceful Parent, Happy Kids: How to Stop Yelling and Start Connecting* (New York: Perigee Books, 2012), 39.
2. Vivek Murthy, *Together: The Healing Power of Human Connection in a Sometimes Lonely World.* (HarperCollins Publishers, 2020), 8.
3. Kerstin Gerst-Emerson and Jayani Jayawardhana, "Loneliness as a Public Health Issue: The Impact of Loneliness on Health Care Utilization among Older Adults," *American Journal of Public Health* 105, no. 5 (May 2015): 1013–19, doi.org/10.2105/ajph .2014.302427.
4. Keziah Weir, "The Charming Billie Eilish," *Vanity Fair*, January 25, 2021, vanityfair.com/style/2021/01/the-charming-billie -eilish-march-cover.
5. Brené Brown, *Dare to Lead: Brave Work, Tough Conversations, Whole Hearts* (New York: Random House, 2018), 42.
6. Robin Dunbar, *How Many Friends Does One Person Need?: Dunbar's Number and Other Evolutionary Quirks.* (Cambridge, MA: Harvard University Press, 2010).
7. Murthy, *Together*, 8.

Chapter 7: The Pillar of Balance

1. "Alcohol and Cancer," Center for Disease Control and Prevention, 2019, cdc.gov/cancer/alcohol/index.htm.
2. Tigershark [pseud], "Origin of H.A.L.T.," *The Road of Happy Destiny* (blog), January 6, 2010, theroadofhappydestiny .blogspot.com/search/label/H.A.L.T.
3. A. H. Maslow, "A Theory of Human Motivation," *Psychological Review* 50, no. 4 (1943): 370, doi.org/10.1037/h0054346.
4. Julianne Holt-Lunstad et al., "Loneliness and Social Isolation as Risk Factors for Mortality: A Meta-Analytic Review," *Perspectives on Psychological Sciences* 10, no. 10 (March 23, 2015): 227–37, scholarsarchive.byu.edu/facpub/1996.

5. Arianna Huffington, *The Sleep Revolution: Transforming Your Life, One Night at a Time* (London: W. H. Allen, 2016).

6. Agnese Mariotti, "The Effects of Chronic Stress on Health: New Insights into the Molecular Mechanisms of Brain–Body Communication," *Future Science OA* 1, no. 3 (November 2015), doi.org/10.4155/fso.15.21.

7. Michael S. Pollard, Joan S. Tucker, and Harold D. Green, "Changes in Adult Alcohol Use and Consequences during the COVID-19 Pandemic in the US," *JAMA Network Open* 3, no. 9 (September 29, 2020), doi.org/10.1001/jamanetworkopen .2020.22942.

8. Whitney Wharton et al., "Neurobiological Underpinnings of the Estrogen-Mood Relationship," *Current Psychiatry Reviews* 8, no. 3 (June 1, 2012): 247–56, doi.org/10.2174 /157340012800792957.

9. Brené Brown, *Rising Strong: How the Ability to Reset Transforms the Way We Live, Love, Parent, and Lead* (New York: Random House, 2017).

10. Susan Cain, *Quiet: The Power of Introverts in a World That Can't Stop Talking* (New York: Crown Publishers, 2012).

Chapter 8: The Pillar of Process

1. Joe Dispenza, *Breaking the Habit of Being Yourself: How to Lose Your Mind and Create a New One* (Carlsbad, CA: Hay House, 2016).

2. Amir Levine and Rachel Heller, *Attached: The New Science of Adult Attachment and How It Can Help You Find—and Keep— Love* (New York: TarcherPerigee, 2011).

3. Gabor Maté and Peter Levine, *In the Realm of Hungry Ghosts: Close Encounters with Addiction* (Berkeley: North Atlantic Books, 2010), 36.

4. Vincent J. Felitti et al., "Relationship of Childhood Abuse and Household Dysfunction to Many of the Leading Causes of Death in Adults," *American Journal of Preventive Medicine* 14, no. 4 (May 1998): 245–58, doi.org/10.1016/s0749-3797(98) 00017-8.

5. Bessel van der Kolk, *The Body Keeps the Score: Brain, Mind, and Body in the Healing of Trauma* (New York: Penguin Books, 2015), 53.

6. Felitti et al., "Relationship of Childhood Abuse," 245.
7. Donna Jackson Nakazawa, *Childhood Disrupted: How Your Biography Becomes Your Biology, and How You Can Heal* (New York: Atria Books, 2015).
8. van der Kolk, *The Body Keeps the Score*, 53.
9. Peter A. Levine and Ann Frederick, *Waking the Tiger—Healing Trauma: The Innate Capacity to Transform Overwhelming Experiences* (Berkeley: North Atlantic Books, 1997).
10. Levine and Frederick, *Waking the Tiger*, 34.
11. Russell Brand, "Vulnerability & Power | Brené Brown & Russell Brand," *Under the Skin*, youtube.com/watch?v=SM1ckkGwqZI.
12. Dawson Church et al., "Guidelines for the Treatment of PTSD Using Clinical EFT (Emotional Freedom Techniques)," *Healthcare* 6, no. 4 (December 12, 2018), doi.org/10.3390/healthcare6040146.
13. van der Kolk, *The Body Keeps the Score*, 67.

Chapter 9: The Pillar of Growth

1. Veronica Valli, *Why You Drink and How to Stop: Journey to Freedom* (US: Ebby Publishing, 2013), 39.
2. Nicole LaPera, "The Holistic Psychologist," YouTube, 2020, youtube.com/watch?v=U3VFzlykm3s&t=148s.
3. Lynn Matti, *5 Weeks to Self-Confidence: A Guide to Confronting Your Inner Critic & Controlling Your Relationship with Your Thoughts* (Emeryville, CA: Rockridge Press, 2019), 47.
4. Glennon Doyle, *Untamed* (New York: The Dial Press, 2020), 57.
5. Eckhart Tolle, *A New Earth: Awakening to Your Life's Purpose* (New York: Plume, 2016), 129.
6. Gay Hendricks, *The Big Leap: Conquer Your Hidden Fear and Take Life to the Next Level* (New York: HarperCollins, 2010), 63.
7. Kelly Ruta, personal communication, 2020.

Conclusion

1. *A Royal Hangover*, directed by Arthur Cauty, DVD (UK: Journeyman Pictures, 2014).
2. Arthur Cauty, personal communication, 2014.
3. Ronald C. Kessler et al., "Patterns and Predictors of Treatment

Seeking after Onset of a Substance Use Disorder," *Archives of General Psychiatry* 58, no. 11 (November 1, 2001): 1065, doi .org/10.1001/archpsyc.58.11.1065.

BIBLIOGRAPHY

Boden, Joseph M., and David M. Fergusson. "Alcohol and Depression." *Addiction* 106, no. 5 (March 7, 2011): 906–14. doi.org/10.1111/j.1360-0443.2010.03351.x.

Brand, Russell. "Vulnerability & Power | Brené Brown & Russell Brand." *Under the Skin.* YouTube, June 23, 2019. youtube.com/watch?v=SM1ckkGwqZI.

Brown, Brené. *Dare to Lead: Brave Work, Tough Conversations, Whole Hearts.* New York: Random House, 2018.

Brown, Brené. *Rising Strong: How the Ability to Reset Transforms the Way We Live, Love, Parent, and Lead.* New York: Random House, 2017.

Cain, Susan. *Quiet: The Power of Introverts in a World That Can't Stop Talking.* New York: Crown Publishers, 2012.

A Royal Hangover. DVD. Directed by Arthur Cauty. UK: Journeyman Pictures, 2014.

CDC (Centers for Disease Control and Prevention). "Alcohol and Cancer." 2019. cdc.gov/cancer/alcohol/index.htm.

Church, Dawson, Peta Stapleton, Phil Mollon, David Feinstein, Elizabeth Boath, David Mackay, and Rebecca Sims. "Guidelines for the Treatment of PTSD Using Clinical EFT (Emotional Freedom Techniques)." *Healthcare* 6, no. 4 (December 12, 2018). doi.org/10.3390/healthcare6040146.

Clapp, Peter, Sanjiv V. Bhave, and Paula L. Hoffman. "How Adaptation of the Brain to Alcohol Leads to Dependence: A Pharmacological Perspective." *Alcohol Research & Health: The Journal of the National Institute on Alcohol Abuse and Alcoholism* 31, no.4 (2008): 310–39. pubmed.ncbi.nlm.nih.gov/20729980/.

Damasio, Antonio R. Feeling Our Emotions. Interview by Manuela Lenzen. *Scientific American*, April 1, 2005. scientificamerican.com/article/feeling-our-emotions/.

Dispenza, Joe. *Breaking the Habit of Being Yourself: How to Lose Your Mind and Create a New One*. Carlsbad, CA: Hay House, 2016.

Doyle, Glennon. *Untamed*. New York: The Dial Press, 2020.

Dunbar, Robin. *How Many Friends Does One Person Need?: Dunbar's Number and Other Evolutionary Quirks*. Cambridge, MA: Harvard University Press, 2010.

Felitti, Vincent J., Robert F. Anda, Dale Nordenberg, David F. Williamson, Alison M. Spitz, Valerie Edwards, Mary P. Koss, and James S. Marks. "Relationship of Childhood Abuse and Household Dysfunction to Many of the Leading Causes of Death in Adults." *American Journal of Preventive Medicine* 14, no. 4 (May 1998): 245–58. doi.org/10.1016/s0749-3797(98)00017-8.

Freimuth, Marilyn, Sandy Moniz, and Shari R. Kim. "Clarifying Exercise Addiction: Differential Diagnosis, Co-Occurring Disorders, and Phases of Addiction." *International Journal of Environmental Research and Public Health* 8, no. 10 (October 8, 2011): 4069–81. doi.org/10.3390/ijerph8104069.

Gerst-Emerson, Kerstin, and Jayani Jayawardhana. "Loneliness as a Public Health Issue: The Impact of Loneliness on Health Care Utilization among Older Adults." *American Journal of*

Public Health 105, no. 5 (May 2015): 1013–19. doi.org/10
.2105/ajph.2014.302427.

Grisel, Judith. *Never Enough: The Neuroscience and Experience of Addiction*. New York: Anchor Books, 2020.

Hardy, Benjamin. *Willpower Doesn't Work: Discover the Hidden Keys to Success*. Hachette Book Group, 2019.

Hendricks, Gay. *The Big Leap: Conquer Your Hidden Fear and Take Life to the Next Level*. New York: HarperCollins, 2010.

Holt-Lunstad, Julianne, Timothy Smith, Mark Baker, Tyler Harris, and David Stephenson. "Loneliness and Social Isolation as Risk Factors for Mortality: A Meta-Analytic Review." *Faculty Publications*, March 23, 2015. scholarsarchive.byu.edu/facpub/1996.

Huffington, Ariana. *The Sleep Revolution: Transforming Your Life, One Night at a Time*. London: W. H. Allen, 2016.

Hyman, Steven E., Robert C. Malenka, and Eric J. Nestler. "Neural Mechanisms of Addiction: The Role of Reward-Related Learning and Memory." *Annual Review of Neuroscience* 29, no. 1 (July 21, 2006): 565–98. doi.org/10 .1146/annurev.neuro.29.051605.113009.

Iwamoto, Derek Kenji, Alice Cheng, Christina S. Lee, Stephanie Takamatsu, and Derrick Gordon. "'Man-Ing' up and Getting Drunk: The Role of Masculine Norms, Alcohol Intoxication and Alcohol-Related Problems among College Men." *Addictive Behaviors* 36, no. 9 (September, 2011). doi.org/10.1016/j.addbeh.2011.04.005.

Jack, Rachael, Oliver G. B. Garrod, and Philippe G. Schyns. "Dynamic Facial Expressions of Emotion Transmit an Evolving Hierarchy of Signals over Time." *Current Biology* 24, no. 2 (January 20, 2014): 187–92. doi.org/10.1016/j.cub.2013.11.064.

Kessler, Ronald C., Sergio Aguilar-Gaxiola, Patricia A. Berglund, Jorge I. Caraveo-Anduaga, David J. DeWit, Whelly F. Greenfield, Bhodan Kolody, Mark Olfson, and William A. Vega. "Patterns and Predictors of Treatment Seeking after Onset of a Substance Use Disorder." *Archives of General Psychiatry* 58, no. 11 (November 1, 2001): 1065–71. doi.org /10.1001/archpsyc.58.11.1065.

Lennox, Jemma, Carol Emslie, Helen Sweeting, and Antonia Lyons. "The Role of Alcohol in Constructing Gender and Class Identities among Young Women in the Age of Social Media." *The International Journal of Drug Policy* 58 (2018): 13–21. doi.org/10.1016.j.drugpo.2018.04.009.

Levine, Amir and Rachel Heller. *Attached: The New Science of Adult Attachment and How It Can Help You Find—and Keep—Love*. New York: TarcherPerigee, 2011.

Levine, Peter A., and Ann Frederick. *Waking the Tiger—Healing Trauma: The Innate Capacity to Transform Overwhelming Experiences*. Berkeley: North Atlantic Books, 1997.

Lin, Tzu-Wei, and Yu-Min Kuo. "Exercise Benefits Brain Function: The Monoamine Connection." *Brain Sciences* 3, no. 1 (January 11, 2013): 39–53. doi.org/doi:10.3390 /brainsci3010039.

Mariotti, Agnese. "The Effects of Chronic Stress on Health: New Insights into the Molecular Mechanisms of Brain–Body Communication." *Future Science OA* 1, no. 3 (November 2015). doi.org/10.4155/fso.15.21.

Markham, Laura. *Peaceful Parent, Happy Kids: How to Stop Yelling and Start Connecting*. New York: Perigee Books, 2012.

Maslow, A. H. "A Theory of Human Motivation." *Psychological Review* 50, no. 4 (1943): 370–96. doi.org/10.1037 /h0054346.

Maté, Gabor and Peter Levine. *In the Realm of Hungry Ghosts: Close Encounters with Addiction.* Berkeley: North Atlantic Books, 2010.

Matti, Lynn. *5 Weeks to Self-Confidence: A Guide to Confronting Your Inner Critic & Controlling Your Relationship with Your Thoughts.* Emeryville, CA: Rockridge Press, 2019.

McGonigal, Kelly. *The Joy of Movement: How Exercise Helps Us Find Happiness, Hope, Connection, and Courage.* New York: Avery, 2019.

Mobbs, Dean, Cindy C. Hagan, Tim Dalgleish, Brian Silston, and Charlotte Prevost. "The Ecology of Human Fear: Survival Optimization and the Nervous System." *Frontiers in Neuroscience*, March 18, 2015. doi.org/10.3389/fnins.2015 .00055.

Mukherjee, Sukhes. "Alcoholism and Its Effects on the Central Nervous System." *Current Neurovascular Research* 10, no. 3 (2013): 256–62. doi.org/10.2174/15672026113109990004.

Murthy, Vivek. *Together: The Healing Power of Human Connection in a Sometimes Lonely World.* HarperCollins Publishers, 2020.

Nakazawa, Donna Jackson. *Childhood Disrupted: How Your Biography Becomes Your Biology and How You Can Heal.* New York: Atria Books, 2015.

Obama, Michelle. *Becoming.* London: Viking, 2018.

Pollard, Michael S., Joan S. Tucker, and Harold D. Green. "Changes in Adult Alcohol Use and Consequences during the COVID-19 Pandemic in the US." *JAMA Network Open* 3, no. 9 (September 29, 2020). doi.org/10.1001 /jamanetworkopen.2020.22942.

Roxo, Marcelo R., Paulo R. Franceschini, Carlos Zubaran, Fabrício D. Kleber, and Josemir W. Sander. "The Limbic System Conception and Its Historical Evolution." *The*

Scientific World Journal 11, no. 11 (2011): 2427–40. doi.org /10.1100/2011/157150.

Russett, Jill Lynne. "Women's Perceptions of High Risk Drinking: Understanding Binge Drinking in a Gender Biased Setting." W&M ScholarWorks (website), 2008. dx .doi.org/doi:10.25774/w4-aygt-cb32.

Tigershark [pseud]. "Origin of H.A.L.T." *The Road of Happy Destiny* (blog). January 6, 2010. theroadofhappydestiny .blogspot.com/search/label/H.A.L.T.

Tolle, Eckhart. *A New Earth: Awakening to Your Life's Purpose.* New York: Plume, 2016.

Valli, Veronica. *Why You Drink and How to Stop: Journey to Freedom.* US: Ebby Publishing, 2013.

van der Kolk, Bessel. *The Body Keeps the Score: Brain, Mind and Body in the Healing of Trauma.* New York: Penguin Books, 2015.

Weir, Keziah. "The Charming Billie Eilish." *Vanity Fair,* January 25, 2021. vanityfair.com/style/2021/01/the -charming-billie-eilish-march-cover.

Wharton, Whitney, Carey E. Gleason, Olson Sandra, Cynthia M. Carlsson, and Sanjay Asthana. "Neurobiological Underpinnings of the Estrogen-Mood Relationship." *Current Psychiatry Reviews* 8, no. 3 (June 1, 2012): 247–56. doi.org /10.2174/157340012800792957.

Whitaker, Holly. *Quit Like a Woman: The Radical Choice to Not Drink in a Culture Obsessed with Alcohol.* London: Bloomsbury, 2021.

ABOUT THE AUTHOR

Veronica has been continuously sober since May 2, 2000. After years of binge drinking, drug use, and mental health problems like depression and anxiety she finally realized that she couldn't use alcohol as a crutch anymore and stopped drinking forever. At twenty-seven years old she thought her life was over and would be dull and gray without alcohol. How wrong she was.

Veronica trained and worked as a clinical psychotherapist in the UK and was accredited by the British Association of Counselling and Psychotherapy. She has started rehab centers and worked in the criminal justice system and government policy. After relocating to the US, she began work as a sober coach and created the Soberful program. As the cohost of the successful *Soberful* podcast with Chip Somers, she reaches a global audience with her positive message about sobriety.

Veronica lives on Lake Tahoe in Nevada with her two sons, husband, and dog.

Free Facebook group: Soberful
Instagram: @veronicajvalli
Website: Soberful.com and Veronicavalli.com
YouTube: Veronica Valli

ABOUT SOUNDS TRUE

Sounds True is a multimedia publisher whose mission is to inspire and support personal transformation and spiritual awakening. Founded in 1985 and located in Boulder, Colorado, we work with many of the leading spiritual teachers, thinkers, healers, and visionary artists of our time. We strive with every title to preserve the essential "living wisdom" of the author or artist. It is our goal to create products that not only provide information to a reader or listener but also embody the quality of a wisdom transmission.

For those seeking genuine transformation, Sounds True is your trusted partner. At SoundsTrue.com you will find a wealth of free resources to support your journey, including exclusive weekly audio interviews, free downloads, interactive learning tools, and other special savings on all our titles.

To learn more, please visit SoundsTrue.com/freegifts or call us toll-free at 800.333.9185.